CANCER TREATMENT RESEARCH

DEVELOPMENTS IN ONCOLOGY
VOLUME 2

Previously published in this series:

1. F.J. Cleton and J.W.I.M. Simons, eds. Genetic Origins of Tumor Cells
   ISBN 90-247-2272-1

CANCER TREATMENT RESEARCH

edited by

JOSEPH AISNER
Division of Cancer Treatment
Baltimore, Maryland, U.S.A.

and

PAUL CHANG
Good Samaritan Hospital
Baltimore, Maryland, U.S.A.

1980

MARTINUS NIJHOFF PUBLISHERS
THE HAGUE / BOSTON / LONDON

Distributors:

for the United States and Canada
Kluwer Boston, Inc.
160 Cld Derby Street
Hingham, MA 02043
USA

for all other countries
Kluwer Academic Publishers Group
Distribution Center
P.O. Box 322
3300 AH Dordrecht
The Netherlands

Library of Congress Cataloging in Publication Data CIP

Main entry under title:

Cancer treatment research.

    (Developments in oncology; v.2)

1. Cancer.
I. Aisner, Joseph. II. Chang, Paul.
III. Series (dnlm: 1. Neoplasms-therapy.
2. Research. W1 DE 998N V.2 QZ266 C2195)

RC 270.8.C39   616.99'4   80-11399

ISBN 90-247-2358-2

PRINTED IN THE NETHERLANDS

TABLE OF CONTENTS

Chapter 1:   NEW APPROACHES TO THE DIAGNOSIS AND CLASSIFICATION
             OF THE NON-HODGKIN'S LYMPHOMAS
             Elaine S. Jaffe, Raul C. Braylan, Koji Nanba and Costan W. Berard

Chapter 2:   STAGING AND TREATMENT OF NON-HODGKIN'S
             LYMPHOMAS
             Charles H. Diggs

STAGING OF NON-HODGKIN'S LYMPHOMAS

Chapter 3:   CURRENT ISSUES IN THE MANAGEMENT OF PATIENTS
           WITH HODGKIN'S DISEASE
           Peter H. Wiernik

Chapter 6: CARCINOMA OF THE THYROID
            Stephen C. Schimpff

Chapter 7: COMPUTED TOMOGRAPHY IN THE EVALUATION OF
            ABDOMINAL MALIGNANCY
            David H. Stephens and Patrick F. Sheedy, II

Chapter 8:   MANAGEMENT OF GASTRIC AND PANCREATIC CANCER
              J.J. Gullo, M. Citron, F.P. Smith, J.S. Macdonald and P.S. Schein

GASTRIC CARCINOMA

CANCER OF THE PANCREAS

Chapter 11:   BREAST PARENCHYMAL PATTERNS ON MAMMOGRAPHY
               AND THEIR RELATIONSHIP TO CARCINOMA
               John N. Wolfe

Chapter 12:   INITIAL MANAGEMENT OF CARCINOMA OF THE BREAST
               WITH RADIATION THERAPY INSTEAD OF MASTECTOMY
               Leonard R. Prosnitz

Chapter 13:   THE SURGICAL TREATMENT OF PRIMARY BREAST
               CANCER
               Richard G. Margolese

Chapter 14: CLINICAL APPLICATIONS OF CELL KINETICS TO
CHEMOTHERAPY OF HUMAN MALIGNANCY
Alvin M. Mauer

Chapter 15: ADJUVANT THERAPY IN CHILDHOOD NEOPLASMS -
AN OVERVIEW
W. W. Sutow

Chapter 16:   AN OVERVIEW OF ADJUVANT THERAPY IN MAN

                    Emil J. Freireich

Chapter 17:   AN OVERVIEW OF UNCONVENTIONAL (FRAUDULENT)

                    TREATMENTS OF CANCER

                    Daniel S. Martin

INTRODUCTION

In recent years the field of cancer treatment has been burgeoning with ever expanding interest and commitments to research and therapy. Besides the large number of specialty journals and publications devoted to cancer related fields, nearly every general medical journal contains one or more articles related to cancer treatment and research. Another example of this expanding commitment and interest is reflected in the Internal Medicine subspecialty of Medical Oncology which, since its recognition as a subspecialty in 1973, has become the secondmost populated subspecialty, second only to cardiology. This burgeoning interest and commitment is obviously appropriate in view of the prevalence and incidence of the various cancers. These diseases constitute, after all, some of the most important and devastating problems of civilized man.

It has been particularly gratifying to those involved with cancer research and therapy to observe the increasing interest in these diseases being translated into real improvements in patient care - improvements in length of survival, improvements in quality of survival, and improvements in palliative care. One need only look at Hodgkin's disease to observe the high rate of cure now routinely obtained whereas, in the past, many patients' disease continued to progress with fatal consequences. Some of these improvements came about through better staging techniques, and other improvements, as will be discussed in the chapter on Hodgkin's, came about from the application of early chemotherapy. Further research in Hodgkin's disease is still going on in order to improve results and decrease treatment related complications.

Another example of the improvements derived in recent years from ongoing treatment research studies has been the realization of improved survival from the application of early or "adjuvant" treatment of micrometastases. Based on solid evidence in the animal tumor systems, the early multimodal treatment of bulk and micrometastatic disease has led to marked improvements in survival of patients with Wilms' tumor, pediatric rhabdomyosarcoma, and osteosarcoma as well as breast cancer. With the principle and the concepts of early treatment of micrometastases firmly established, new studies are being rapidly carried forward on a variety of diseases such as gastric cancer in which active therapy of advanced disease has been identified. In other tumors, such as pancreatic cancer, active drugs and combinations are being sought in the advanced stage of the disease with the aim of eventually applying such active drugs or treatment modalities earlier in the course of the disease.

Parallel to such advances in therapy, a large effort at earlier diagnosis is being made in order to institute therapy of cancer at its earliest and most potentially curable state. Such diagnostic efforts would also lead to methods which could help evaluate, measure and follow difficult tumors. Thus newer methods or new applications of established methods (such as those discussed in the chapters on mammography) allow for the identification of early cancers. Other techniques such as CAT scans could allow for the identification, measurement and sequential follow-up of difficult tumors such as pancreatic carcinoma, in which measurable disease has been a stumbling block in the past for evaluating potentially active agents or treatments.

This volume, derived in part from a past continuing education symposium held by the Baltimore Cancer Research Program, has brought together a group of medical investigators involved in cancer research to review their respective areas from the standpoint of actual and anticipated advances in cancer treatment. The spectrum of the material thus ranges from basic medical and scientific information necessary for staging and therapy (as discussed in the chapters on non-Hodgkin's lymphomas) to the anticipated changes within the next decade. The chapters on head and neck cancers deal with treatment for this group of cancers for which newer agents and treatment approaches, such as combined modality therapy or pre-operative application of chemotherapy, will hopefully lead to marked improvements. The discussion of abdominal CAT scans naturally leads into discussion of intra-abdominal cancers of the stomach, pancreas and bladder. The discussions of mammography for the early detection of breast cancer lead into the chapters dealing with newer approaches for the primary management of breast cancer with either radiotherapy or lesser surgical procedures. The chapters on the early therapy of micrometastases review the striking success seen in the pediatric tumors as well as the principles involved in the design and management of "adjuvant" treatment programs. Other discussions include cell kinetics and their use in predicting optimal application of therapy, and a discussion of unconventional treatments in cancer. With these reviews of a wide spectrum of cancer diagnosis and treatment, we hope to present a very large body of information in a relatively compact and easily digested format.

Joseph Aisner

Paul Chang

NEW APPROACHES TO THE DIAGNOSIS AND CLASSIFICATION OF THE NON-HODGKIN'S LYMPHOMAS

Elaine S. Jaffe, M.D., Raul C. Braylan, M.D.,
Koji Nanba, M.D., Costan W. Berard, M.D.
National Cancer Institute
National Institutes of Health
Bethesda, Maryland

INTRODUCTION

Malignant lymphomas have been traditionally classified morphologically. The classification published by Rappaport in 1966 (1), with minor modifications (2,3), has been the one most widely employed for clinicopathologic studies (table 1).

Table 1

CLASSIFICATION OF NON-HODGKIN'S LYMPHOMAS (1-3)

Nodular

        Lymphocytic, poorly differentiated
        Mixed lymphocytic-histiocytic
        Histiocytic

Diffuse

        Lymphocytic, well differentiated
        Lymphocytic, intermediate differentiation
        Lymphocytic, poorly differentiated
        Mixed lymphocytic-histiocytic
        Histiocytic
        Undifferentiated (Burkitt's type)
        Undifferentiated, pleomorphic (non-Burkitt's)
        Lymphoblastic

However, with the recognition of malignant lymphomas as neoplastic disorders of the immune system, a new functional approach has been undertaken for the classification and understanding of these tumors. Immunological knowledge and techniques have been brought to bear on clinical and pathological problems. For example, the concepts of homing and "traffic" of normal lymphocytes help to explain the patterns of spread of these tumors. Likewise, the immunological deficits manifested by these patients relate to which component of the immune system is affected by neoplasia. One major area of investigation which typifies this approach has been the study of the neoplastic cells themselves, both for the presence of cell surface markers as well as in functional assays (table 2).

Table 2

TECHNIQUES USED IN THE INVESTIGATION
OF LYMPHORETICULAR MALIGNANCIES

1. Membrane bound immunoglobulins - SIg
   individual light and heavy chains
   in vitro synthesis
2. Intracytoplasmic immunoglobulin
   immunofluorescence
   immunoperoxidase
3. Complement receptors - EAC rosettes
4. Receptors for cytophilic antibody - IgGEA rosettes
5. Spontaneous SRBC binding - E rosettes
6. In vitro phagocytosis
7. Cytochemical markers
   "non-specific" esterases
   acid phosphatase
   beta-glucuronidase
   alkaline phosphatase
8. Terminal deoxynucleotidyl transferase (TdT)
9. In vitro culture of neoplastic cells

By analogy with normal cells, many of the tumors have been classified according to their presumptive cells of origin: T lymphocyte, B lymphocyte, or monocyte-macrophage (table 3).

Table 3

SUMMARY OF CELL SURFACE MARKERS IN LYMPHORETICULAR MALIGNANCIES

Well-differentiated lymphocytic malignancies	B lymphocytic
Chronic lymphocytic leukemia	
Well-differentiated lymphocytic lymphoma	
Waldenstrom's macroglobulinemia	
Lymphocytic lymphoma, intermediate	B lymphocyitc
Nodular (Follicular) lymphoma	B lymphocytic
Burkitt's lymphoma	B lymphocytic
Mycosis fungoides	T lymphocytic
Sezary syndrome	
Lymphoblastic lymphoma	T lymphocytic
Acute lymphoblastic leukemia (25%)	
Histiocytic lymphomas	Heterogenous
Malignant histiocytosis	Histiocytic

LYMPHOMAS ORIGINATING FROM B LYMPHOCYTES

Most non-Hodgkin's lymphomas in adults appear to be of B lymphocytic origin. However, different B-cell populations display subtle variations in their surface markers and have thus permitted the assignment of some lymphomas to particular subpopulations. The cells of the lymphoid follicle are characterized by abundant surface immunoglobulin (SIg) and avid complement receptors, but as a B cell differentiates towards a plasma cell there is a loss of both of these surface membrane markers. Of course, intermediate stages also are present in which SIg is reduced in density and complement receptors are sparse.

Nodular lymphomas are cytologically and immunologically tumors composed of follicular B lymphocytes (4-6). These tumors are a major category of non-Hodgkin's lymphomas in adults, representing approximately 50% of all cases. Clinically these tumors are most often generalized at diagnosis, presenting as stage III or IV disease. Peripheral lymph node groups are frequently involved as are mesenteric nodes, bone marrow and liver (7). However, in spite of its widespread dissemination, this disease may be compatible with relatively long survival, even without aggressive therapy (8). This favorable prognosis appears to be particularly true of the nodular lymphomas of poorly differentiated lymphocytic type, in which the tendency of these tumors to disseminate seems related to the capacity of the neoplastic lymphoid cells to migrate or home like normal lymphoid cells (9). The large cells or "histiocytes" within these tumors represent the proliferative component and, when such cells are present in increased numbers, as in nodular lymphomas of mixed or histiocytic type, the disease is associated with a more aggressive clinical course (10), especially if one does not achieve a complete remission.

Cytologically nodular lymphomas reflect the composition of a normal germinal center (11-12). Immunologically, these tumors also have the characteristics of follicular B lymphocytes. We have previously published on the surface membrane markers of nodular lymphomas and have shown avid complement receptors on the neoplastic cells, also a feature of normal follicular B lymphocytes (4). Other authors have found easily detectable SIg, usually of the IgM class with or without IgD (5,6). Our studies have now been expanded to include a total of 49 specimens from 36 patients and earlier observations have been confirmed (table 4). Strong binding of erythrocyte-antibody complement rosettes (EAC), both in suspensions and on frozen sections, was seen in 48 of the 49. Thirty-two studied for SIg had bright staining of the neoplastic cells in all but one. Fifteen were evaluated for individual light and heavy chains, i.e., k and λ, as well as IgM, IgG and IgA. In all instances the SIg was monoclonal with only a single light chain. IgM was the heavy chain in 13 of the 15. Only kappa light chains were found in two, but these were not studied for IgD. Two of five specimens studied for IgD were positive and in one of these both IgD and IgM were identified with only kappa light chains. The coexistence of surface bound IgD and IgM has been reported in other B lymphocytic tumors, most commonly in chronic lymphocytic leukemia, and does not contradict the monoclonality of these neoplasms (13). When an anti-idiotypic antibody was prepared, the IgD and IgM were shown to be of the same idiotype and even to share the same antibody specificity.

Table 4

NODULAR (FOLLICULAR) LYMPHOMAS

Summary of Surface Markers

49 Specimens from 36 Individuals

EAC	48/49	Strong Rosettes	
SIg	31/32	Bright Staining	
	Monoclonal		15/15
	IgM (with either K or λ)		13/15
	IgD (with and without IgM)		2/5
E	38% ($\overline{M}$) No demonstration on neoplastic cells		

Abbreviations: EAC, erythrocyte-antibody complement rosettes; SIg, surface immunoglobulin; E, rosette formation with unsensitized sheep erythrocytes; $\overline{M}$, mean.

LOCALIZATION OF T CELLS IN NODULAR LYMPHOMAS

Nodes

The percentages of T cells (E rosette forming cells) in lymph nodes involved by nodular lymphoma are somewhat variable but often higher than initially expected. In our series lymph nodes from untreated patients contained a mean of $41 \pm 13\%$ E rosette forming cells (ERFC) (table 5). The mean percentage of ERFC in recurrences after therapy was somewhat lower ($34 \pm 19\%$). At present there is no evidence to indicate that these T cells are part of the neoplastic process, since cytologically they are invariably normal. From earlier studies we had speculated that the T cells were probably located in the internodular stroma, since these areas were populated by predominantly normal appearing lymphocytes. Furthermore, with progressive replacement of the nodal parenchyma by tumor, the percentage of ERFC was reduced (4). However, the lack of a method for identifying T cells in sections precluded their precise localization.

Table 5

FREQUENCY AND DISTRIBUTION OF LYMPHOCYTES
IN NODULAR LYMPHOMAS

	Before Therapy	After Therapy
% E	Lymph nodes (11) M 41±13	Lymph nodes (12) M 34±19
	Spleens (3) M 42±9	Spleens (4) M 27±12
E in Frozen Sections	Lymph Nodes 8/11 nodular or perinodular	Lymph nodes 7/12 nodular or perinodular
	3/11 internodular	5/12 internodular
	Spleens 3/3 perifollicular	Spleens 3/4 perifollicular

We have subsequently applied to nodular lymphomas the method of Tonder et al. for the identification of ERFC in frozen tissue sections (14). The method was performed according to Tonder with slight modification. Sheep red blood cells (SRBC) were pretreated with neuraminadase (E_N) as previously described (15). The frozen sections were incubated for 18 hours at $4^{\circ}C$ with a solution of 0.5% E_N in 20% heat-inactivated fetal calf serum previously absorbed with SRBC. After incubation the sections were inverted for 30 min. at $4^{\circ}C$ and read without fixation. The sections were examined in parallel with serial frozen sections stained with hematoxylin and eosin. Twenty-three lymph nodes involved by nodular lymphoma of either poorly differentiated lymphocytic type (NPDL) or mixed cell type were studied. Eleven nodes were obtained prior to any therapy whereas 12 lymph nodes represented post-therapy recurrences. Seven spleens involved by NPDL were studied, three before therapy and four after therapy. Control tissues included normal or reactive lymph nodes and spleens, normal thymus, and lymph nodes involved by chronic lymphocytic leukemia of B cell type containing negligible T cells.

The tissues studied by the frozen section technique were also studied in suspension and the percent T cells determined. The mean percent ERFC was 41 ± 13 in nodes obtained prior to therapy and 34 ± 19 in the recurrences (table 5). In the spleens the mean percent ERFC was 42 ± 9 before therapy and 27 ± 12 after treatment.

In lymph nodes involved by nodular lymphoma the strongest reactions with E_N were not internodular, as had been anticipated, but within the nodules, particularly at the periphery of the nodules. These perinodular reactions were very striking in the majority of cases. They assumed the configuration of the nodules with a weaker reaction in the central portions. This same localization was present in lymph nodes obtained either before or after therapy. Of eleven lymph nodes obtained prior to therapy, eight showed a nodular or perinodular reaction that was greater than or equal to the internodular reaction. Only three cases showed a negative nodular reaction with the predominant E_N adherence being internodular. The nodular or perinodular reactions were generally less striking in the recurrences but still were evident in seven of twelve cases. In five cases the predominant reactions were internodular and the nodules themselves were negative.

Spleen

The findings were somewhat different in spleens involved by nodular lymphoma. Those areas of the malphighian follicles histologically replaced by neoplastic cells showed only weakly positive reaction. The strongest reactions were at the periphery of the white pulp, an area thought to be normally populated by T cells (16). However, the peripheral T cell reactions in spleens involved by nodular lymphoma were much greater than those in any of the normal spleens studied. These reactions did seem to correlate histologically with a prominent zone of normal lymphocytes and immunoblasts. Only one case failed to show this peripheral white pulp reaction and this case also lacked the hyperplastic features described above.

The strong binding of E_N to the nodules of nodular lymphoma was unexpected and we wanted to confirm that the adherence was due to the interaction of SRBC and T lymphocytes. Control studies appeared to support this conclusion. Very strong reactions were observed between thymocytes in sections and E_N. In contrast, tissues involved by CLL containing few ERFC in suspension showed essentially no binding to frozen sections, with only rare isolated rosettes. Additional controls were performed on tissues involved by nodular lymphoma.

The reaction was shown to be inhibited by trypsinization of the SRBC, a procedure known to inhibit the E rosette phenomenon (15). It was speculated that perhaps the SIg associated with the nodular lymphoma cells was mediating the E binding via antibody activity, but pretreatment of frozen sections with anti-human immunoglobulin did not inhibit the reaction. Furthermore, a strong reaction was also observed in the one case that was SIg-negative. Similar incubations were performed using human and rabbit red cells, since both human and Rhesus monkey but not rabbit red cells have been reported to interact with human T lymphocytes in a manner similar to SRBC (17-20). With human red cells a weak but similar reaction to that observed with SRBC was observed. However, the rabbit red cells did not demonstrate specific patterns of localization.

All of the above evidence indicates the presence of T lymphocytes within the nodules of nodular lymphoma. The significance of this finding is not as yet understood. These cells may well be reactive and not part of the neoplastic clone. On cytocentrifuge preparations, as mentioned above, these ERFC always appear cytologically normal. Furthermore, in patients with prior nodular lymphoma recurring as diffuse histiocytic lymphoma, the percentage of ERFC is almost invariably low as will be seen in table 8 below. Finally, even in those patients wth recurrent nodular disease, the percent ERFC appears slightly reduced. The T cells within the tumors could be part of the host defense since T cell infiltrates have been described in a variety of malignant tumors (21).

Internodular Areas

It is still puzzling that E_N bound relatively poorly to the internodular areas. Histologically these areas are populated by normal-appearing lymphocytes, presumably T cells since they fail to bind EAC. Activated T lymphocytes have been reported to bind E more readily than T cells not stimulated or not actively participating in an immune response (22). This ready binding has been used as the basis for the active-E rosette test (22). It is conceivable that those cells in the internodular areas are an inactive, residual population, which bind E_N poorly. The T cells within the nodules might be immunologically stimulated and thus bind E_N more strongly in the frozen section assay. These tissues were not assayed in suspension for the active-E population. Our studies are preliminary and further work is necessary to determine whether or not there is a correlation between T cell infiltration and other morphologic and/or clinical parameters.

WELL DIFFERENTIATED LYMPHOMAS

The immunologic features of nodular lymphoma cells summarized above can be contrasted with those of the cells of well differentiated lymphoid malignancies. The latter have either a qualitative or quantitative deficiency in complement receptors and poorly express SIg (23). These differences have been related to different B-cell subpopulations in that they support a relationship of the well-differentiated lymphocytic malignancies to the secretory B-cell system (9). In chronic lymphocytic leukemia (CLL) a block in the maturation of B cells into plasma cells seems to occur; clinically these patients may have hypogamma-globulinemia and humoral immune deficiency (24). Is this block in differentiation due to an intrinsic defect in the neoplastic B cells? Some recent evidence indicates that this may not be the case. Fu et al. have recently reported on the defective helper T-cell function of the residual T cells in CLL (25). These T cells in an in vitro assay system fail to subserve a helper function for both neoplastic B cells as well as normal tonsillar B lymphocytes. However, when the neoplastic B cells were co-cultured with normal T cells, they could be induced to differentiate into plasma cells and secrete immunoglobulin. Of course, it is not known if this T cell defect is primary or secondary, and there is no evidence to suggest that the T cells are part of the neoplastic process.

In the context of well differentiated lymphoid malignancies, Waldenstrom's macroglobulinemia represents one step further in the maturation of a medullary cord B cell into a plasma cell. In this disease the cells have both cytoplasmic and surface Ig and of course secretion of IgM occurs with the production of a monoclonal spike. Notably, in this disease, a defect in helper T-cell function was not present (25).

INTERMEDIATE DIFFERENTIATION

Histologic Features

Malignant lymphomas of lymphocytic type of intermediate differentiation (LI) have pathologic features intermediate between those of nodular lymphoma and well differentiated lymphocytic lymphoma (WDL) (2). These tumors usually are diffuse but may have a vaguely nodular pattern. Cytologically there is a population of cells with sparse cytoplasm and nuclei that exhibit a mature clumped chromatin pattern but a range in shape from round to slightly clefted and irregular. Immunologically these tumors also appear intermediate. Table 6 summarizes the data of six cases. All were of B-lymphocytic type. The cells had monoclonal SIg, usually with an IgM heavy chain. Two such cases also had a minority of cells with IgD. One case had surface IgG. The fluorescent staining was easily seen and of intermediate intensity when compared with NPDL and WDL. The cells also had complement receptors and bound EAC relatively well, both in suspension and on frozen tissue sections. The number of ERFC was in general low, lower than in nodular lymphomas, and was in keeping with the diffuse replacement seen histologically. One case (277) was atypical in that the tissues were only focally involved by the neoplastic process. Both lymph nodes and spleen showed extensive non-caseating granulomatous inflammation. This admixed reactive process probably accounts for the high percentage ERFC identified in suspensions (table 6). The details of this case are reported elsewhere (26).

Table 6

LYMPHOCYTIC LYMPHOMAS OF INTERMEDIATE DIFFERENTIATION

Case No.	Tissue	E*	EAC	IgGEA	SIg	Clon.	EAC-FS	ALP
329	LN	16	80	6	80	MDK	++++	+
325	LN	21	64	7	50	Gk	+++	-
311	LN	6	76	16	55	MDk	++	-
275	LN	25	50	7	61	M	++++	-
228	LN	17	85	17	85	Mk+	++	+
	LN	19	86	36	90	MDk	++	+
277	LN	76	18	2	15	Mk	+++	+
	SPL	63	23	16	34	Mk	+++	+

*results are expressed as % positive cells.

+not studied for IgD.

Abbreviations: LN, lymph node; SPL, spleen; Clon., clonality; EAC-FS, rosette formation on frozen tissue sections; IgGEA, rosette formation with IgG coated erythrocytes; ALP, alkaline phosphatase activity.

Histochemical Features

The LI tumors were also studied histochemically for the enzymes mentioned above. In three of six cases the cells had surface alkaline phosphatase (ALP) activity (27) (table 6). This enzyme has also been identified in a small percentage of nodular lymphomas (27), but is rare in lymphomas of other histologic subtypes. In normal lymph nodes ALP is found on the membranes of follicular cuff lymphocytes, but not on lymphoid cells in other areas. LI tumors thus appear histologically, immunologically and histochemically to be truly intermediate between nodular (follicular) lymphomas and WDL. The cells of nodular lymphomas are neoplastic counter-parts of follicular B lymphocytes whereas WDL cells are more closely related to medullary cord B cells. Lymphomas of LI type may derive from B cells of the lymphoid cuff at the margin of follicles and thus manifest features at the interface between nodular lymphomas and WDL.

BURKITT'S LYMPHOMAS

Burkitt's lymphomas represent yet another category of B-cell tumors. Although there are clinical differences between Burkitt's lymphomas in endemic regions of east Africa and those in non-endemic areas around the world, histologically these tumors are indistinguishable (28). Immunologically they are also identical. They are characterized by abundant monoclonal SIg, usually of the IgM class, but complement receptors are identified in only a fraction of the cases, and when present, usually are found on less than 10 percent of the malignant cells (29, 30). However, the selective involvement of germinal centers in partially involved lymph nodes has suggested at least a morphologic link to germinal center B cells. Lukes and Collins cytologically relate the cells of Burkitt's lymphoma to the small non-cleaved cell of the germinal center (11).

LYMPHOMAS OF T-CELL ORIGIN

T-cell tumors are less common than B-cell lymphomas especially in the adult age group. Furthermore, the ability to identify subpopulations of T cells also is limited. Mycosis fungoides and Sezary's syndrome represent one category of T-cell malignancy (31,31), and functional studies have shown that Sezary cells may in some cases act as helper T cells (33).

Lymphoblastic Lymphomas

Lymphoblastic lymphomas are a relatively recently recognized pathologic entity (3). These tumors occur most often in adolescents and young adults, but can occur at any age. Males are much more frequently affected than females. The frequent association of this tumor with an anterior mediastinal mass at presentation had suggested a relationship to the thymus gland. Indeed, T-cell markers have been identified in a majority of cases and the cells in particular have the surface, cytochemical and biochemical features of immature thymo-cytes (34-37). The high risk of leukemic progression further relates these tumors to a subset of acute lymphoblastic leukemia (ALL), i.e., the 25% of cases of ALL with T-cell markers (38-39).

Table 7 summarizes the immunologic, cytochemical and biochemical features of twelve cases of lymphoblastic lymphoma. Nine of 12 (75%) were males and all but one were 30 or less years of age. Ten of 12 (83%) had anterior mediastinal masses at presentation. In only 6 of 12 cases (50%) did the neoplastic cells have T-cell markers as defined by E rosette formation. It is possible that had these cases been studied for T-cell associated heteroantigens, an additional subset would have been recognized as T-cell in nature. In 5 of 12 cases (42%) complement receptors were identified and in three of these five, complement receptors and sheep erythrocyte receptors coexisted. In no case were other B-cell markers identified. In 4 of 12 cases (33%) no markers were identified. Eight cases were also studied cytochemically for acid phosphatase activity. Some degree of activity was seen in all cases but in general the enzyme activity was intense and punctate in character in only those cases in which the neoplastic cells formed E rosettes. Intense punctate staining for acid phosphatase has also been described in T-cell ALL. The E-negative cases in our series tended to have diffuse multigranular acid phosphatase activity. All cases studied were positive for terminal deoxynucleotidyl transferase (TdT) activity (40).

The heterogeneity of surface markers in these cases is similar to our previously reported experience (36). Conceptually one can relate these tumors to different stages in the maturation of thymic lymphoblasts. As with fetal thymocytes (37), the complement receptor may be a feature of the most primitive cells and this marker is lost as the cells differentiate or mature. Punctate acid phosphatase activity appears to correlate with E rosette formation and TdT activity is present in all cases.

Table 7

LYMPHOBLASTIC LYMPHOMA

Case No.	Age Sex	Med. Mass	Source	E*	EAC	SIg	AP	TdT
87	12F	+	PB	7	85+	8	ND	ND
157	23M	+	PB	10	9	8	ND	ND
162	18M	+	BM	3	4	0	ND	ND
166	22M	+	PB	80+	70+	0	ND	ND
240	19M	+	LN	7	30+	0	+M	+
306	60M	−	Skin	20+	9	0	ND	+
		−	PB	6	3	ND	+M	−
312	18M	+	PF	32+	34+	1	+P	+
344	30F	+	PF	23+	16+	0	+P	+
376	23M	+	PF	63+	NS	0	+P	+
394	22M	+	LN	70+	1	2	+P	+
405	8F	−	Tibia	0	ND	1	+M	+
485	25M	+	BM	3	4	35	+M	ND

*   Results are expressed on % positive cells; + indicates marker identified on neoplastic cells.

M   Multigranular reaction product.

P   Punctate perinuclear reaction product.

Abbreviations: PB, peripheral blood; BM, bone marrow; LN, lymph node; PF, pleural fluid; med., mediastinal mass; ND, not determined; NS, not satisfactory; AP, acid phosphatase; TdT, terminal deoxynucleotidyl transferase.

LARGE CELL LYMPHOMAS

Diffuse "histiocytic" lymphomas have been the subject of relatively few detailed functional studies (41, 42). We have recently completed a study of the membrane surface markers and histochemical profile of 25 large cell malignant lymphomas (table 8). Morphologically 18 were classified as diffuse "histiocytic," five were designated as undifferentiated, pleomorphic (2), and two were called diffuse, mixed cell type. The neoplastic cells were studied in suspension for spontaneous rosette (E) formation with SRBC, receptors for complement (EAC), receptors for cytophilic antibody (IgGEA) and surface immunoglobulins (SIg) (30). Enzyme histochemical techniques on frozen sections, as well as cytochemical reactions

Table 8. MARKERS OF DIFFUSE LARGE CELL, MIXED,

B-Cell	Source	DX	SIg	Clon.	EAC	EA	E
*171	LN	DH	75	ND	14	19	-
*180	LN	DH	92	ND	43	-	-
*181	LN	DH	NS	ND	50	ND	NS
*196	LN	UND	40	ND	80	ND	-
*251	SPL	DH	41	Mk	39	50	-
	LN	DH	45	Mk	64	41	-
*271	PB	DH	85	Mk	-	-	-
*402	LN	DH	90	ND	9	9	-
134	SPL	DH	50	ND	50	-	-
186	BM	DH	95	Mk	-	93	-
293	LN	UND	62	k	32	-	-
296	INT	DH	63	Mk	38	-	-
323	LN	DH	98	Mk	29	-	-
400	PB	DM	84	Mk	-	73	-
T-Cell							
174	LN	DH	-	ND	NS	NS	85
397	LN	UND	-	ND	-	-	41
428	PB	DM	-	ND	-	-	55
444	LN	DH	-	ND	-	-	61
HIST							
298	BONE	DH	-	ND	33	19	-
NULL							
47	LN	DH	ND	ND	-	-	-
91	INT	UND	ND	ND	-	-	-
210	PB	DH	-	ND	-	-	-
349	ASC	UND	-	ND	-	-	-
389	LN	DH	-	ND	-	-	-
418	LN	DH	-	ND	-	ND	-
421	LN	DH	-	-	-	-	-

ˣ Previous diagnosis of nodular (follicular) lymphoma.
Abbreviations: LN, lymph node; SPL, spleen; PB, peripheral blood; BM, bone marrow; INT, intestine; ASC, ascitic fluid; Dx, pathological diagnosis; DH, diffuse histiocytic; UND, diffuse undifferentiated (non-

AND UNDIFFERENTIATED (NON-BURKITT'S) LYMPHOMAS

B-EST	A-EST	AP	BG	TdT	Neoplastic Cell Markers
-	-	-	ND	ND	SIg EAC EA
-	-	-	ND	ND	SIg EAC
-	-	-	ND	ND	EAC
-	-	-	ND	ND	SIg EAC
-	-	-	-	-	SIg EAC EA
-	-	-	-	ND	SIg EAC EA
-	-	-	++	-	SIg BG
-	-	-	-	-	SIg EAC EA
-	-	-	ND	ND	SIG EAC
-	±	±	ND	ND	SIG EA
-	-	-	-	ND	SIg EAC
-	±	+	±	-	SIg EAC AP
-	-	-	-	-	SIg EAC
-	ND	ND	ND	ND	SIg EA
±	++	++	ND	ND	E A-EST,AP
-	-	++	++	-	E AP,BG
-	ND	++	++	ND	E AP,BG
-	-	++	++	ND	E AP,BG
+	++	++	++	ND	EAC EA B-EST,A-EST AP,BG
-	-	-	ND	ND	
-	-	-	ND	-	
-	++	++	ND	ND	A-EST,AP
-	+	+	+	-	A-EST,AP,BG
-	-	-	-	+/-	
-	-	-	-	ND	
-	+	+	ND	ND	A-EST,AP

Burkitt's); DM, diffuse mixed; NS, not satisfactory; ND, not done; Clon., clonality; B-EST, alpha-naphthyl butyrate esterase; A-EST, alpha-naphthyl acetate esterase; AP, acid phosphatase; BG, beta-glucuronidase; TdT, terminal deoxynucleotidyl transferase.

on cytocentrifuge preparations of some cases, were used to identify the following hydrolytic enzymes: acid phosphatase (AP) with and without tartrate, alkaline phosphatase (ALP), B-glucuronidase (BG) and a variety of esterases (EST) including a-naphthyl acetate esterase (A-EST), a-naphthyl butyrate esterase (B-EST), naphthol ASD chloroacetate esterase (ASDC1), and naphthyl ASD acetate esterase (NASDA) with and without NaF inhibition (30,43). The data regarding the immunologic and histochemical features of these cases are summarized in (table 8).

Surface Markers

In 13 of 25 cases (52%) B-lymphocytic markers were identified. However, there was marked variation in the number of markers detected as well as in the percentages of neoplastic cells expressing particular markers. SIg was the most consistent marker, being present in all suitably evaluated cases. In eight cases studied for individual heavy and light chains, IgM and k were identified. Surface bound IgM has also been the most frequent heavy chain class in other B lymphocytic malignancies, including nodular lymphoma (5,6), chronic lymphocytic leukemia (44) and Burkitt's lymphoma (29,30). This finding is not unexpected since IgM is the predominant immunoglobulin class found on normal peripheral blood B lymphocytes (24). In one case only k light chains were identified, without detectable heavy chains. However, this case was not studied for IgD. None of these 13 cases contained significant hydrolytic enzyme activity.

Tumor Overgrowth or Recurrence

Seven of the 25 large cell lymphomas arose in patients with a prior diagnosis of nodular lymphoma and these invariably manifested B-cell markers. Such tumors apparently result from a dedifferentiation or overgrowth of the proliferative element of the neoplasm. A similar phenomenon occurs in blastic transformation of chronic myelogenous leukemia, in which the blasts retain the Ph' chromosome. Identical observations have been reported with other lymphoid neoplasms, i.e., blastic transformation of chronic lymphocytic leukemia (CLL) (45) and large cell malignant lymphomas supervening on CLL (42), so-called Richter's syndrome. In rare instances in which both the antecedent well-differentiated proliferation and the blastic tumor were studied, the membrane bound immunoglobulins were of the same light and heavy chain class supporting the concept that both tumors belonged to one neoplastic clone.

T-Cell Markers

Four of the 25 cases (16%) had T-cell markers. The neoplastic cells formed E rosettes and also had abundant granular activity for acid phosphatase and beta-glucuronidase. Similar enzymatic activity has been reported in other T-cell malignancies such as the Sezary's syndrome (46), chronic lymphocytic leukemia with T-cell markers (47), and lymphoblastic lymphoma (48,49). TdT was absent in the three cases so studied, further evidence that these tumors are distinct from the lymphoblastic lymphomas of T-cell origin. One case (539) was an enlarged cervical lymph node from a 65 year old white male with a history of previously studied Sezary's syndrome, previously studied for lymphocyte surface markers and functional activity. He relapsed with rapidly progressive lymphadenopathy and the lymph node biopsy was diagnosed morphologically as malignant lymphoma, undifferentiated non-Burkitt's type. The neoplastic cells retained T-cell markers and also retained the ability to function as helper cells in an in vitro assay (50).

Histiocytic Origin

One of the 25 cases (4%) (298) had markers consistent with a true histiocytic origin. The cells lacked SIg but formed rosettes with both EAC and IgGEA. In addition, they phagocytosed bound erythrocytes, a phenomenon seen by us only with cells of the monocyte-macrophage series. They also contained abundant hydrolytic enzymes, manifested as diffuse strong cytoplasmic positivity for AP, A-EST, B-G, and NASDA and weak staining for B-EST. Unlike the other cases, this tumor was primary in the bone (clavicle) of a 14 year old boy. The cells were large and pleomorphic with abundant acidophilic cytoplasm. The nuclei were large and often lobulated with prominent eosinophilic nucleoli.

"Null"-Cells

In the remaining seven cases (25%) no immunologic markers were detected; however, two of these cases were not studied for SIg. The neoplastic cells in three cases contained AP and A-EST; one of these was also studied for BG and was positive. However, the staining pattern was not diffuse, as in cells of the monocyte-macrophage series. Rather, the activity was present as discrete punctate dots, in one case restricted to the Golgi zone. This pattern of enzymatic activity is seen in lymphocytes, both normal and neoplastic. It has been reported in T-cell tumors, but T-cell markers were not demonstrable in these cases. One such case (349) was also investigated for and lacked TdT activity. All three cases had plasmacytoid features morphologically, and two studied ultrastructurally contained moderate to abundant amounts of rough endoplasmic reticulum (51,52). Mature plasma cells and myeloma cells are reported to contain AP activity. Unlike these cell types, however, the neoplastic cells lacked detectable intracytoplasmic immunoglobulin. One of the "null" cell cases was studied for TdT both by a biochemical assay (40) and by indirect immunofluorescence (53). Although the biochemical study showed a positive result, this positivity failed to be confirmed by the immunofluorescent study (53). Since, in a series of over 50 cases, this case is the only one in which the immunofluorescent assay failed to confirm the biochemical assay (54), we believe the positivity of this case for TdT must be viewed with caution.

SUMMARY

The study of malignant lymphomas for membrane surface markers and enzyme histochemical features often permits the identification of the cytogeneology of the neoplastic cells. Furthermore, the application of these techniques to frozen tissue sections allows one to observe the interrelationships of various cell types present, both benign and malignant. Recent studies reviewed in this report indicate that most large cell malignant lymphomas (so-called "histiocytic") are of lymphocytic origin, usually of the B-cell type (52%). Tumors composed of neoplastic T-cells are less common (16), and those composed of histiocytes (4%) are quite rare. In 28% no markers were demonstrable. Lymphoblastic lymphomas exhibit some heterogeneity of their membrane surface markers. Receptors for sheep erythrocytes (E) were found in 50% of cases, as were receptors for complement (42%). In 25% of cases these two markers were present simultaneously, and in four cases (33%) neither marker was identified. However, the invariable presence of terminal deoxynucleotidyl transferase activity links all of these tumors to lymphoblasts and suggests that they represent different stages in thymic or T-cell differentiation. Acid-phosphatase activity was also consistently present, but the pattern of activity appeared to correlate with the presence or absence of E rosette formation.

Studies of 49 cases of nodular lymphoma confirm the follicular B-cell nature of the neoplastic cells. Additional studies on the localization of T lymphocytes within these tumors indicate that morphologically normal T cells are also present within the nodules in most cases. These observations suggest that the T lymphocytes although benign, may be functionally interacting with the neoplastic B cells. Well-differentiated lymphocytic malignancies appear to relate to the secretory B-cell system, and may represent blocks at different stages in the differentiation of medullary cord B lymphocytes. Studies of diffuse lymphocytic lymphomas of intermediate differentiation indicate that these B-cell tumors have immunologic features intermediate between follicular lymphomas and well-differentiated lymphocytic malignancies. Cytochemically and immunologically they appear related to follicular cuff lymphocytes.

ACKNOWLEDGEMENT

The authors are grateful to Mrs. Eileen Sussman and Mr. Edward Soban for technical assistance, and to Mrs. Kathleen Erickson for secretarial support, all of the Laboratory of Pathology of the National Cancer Institute.

REFERENCES

1. Rappaport, H, Tumors of the hematopoietic system. In Atlas of Tumor Pathology, Section III, Fascicle *, Armed Forces Institutes of Pathology, Washington, D.C., 1966

2. Berard, CW and RF Dorfman, Histopathology of malignant lymphomas. Clin Hemat 3:39-76, 1974

3. Nathwani, BN, H Kim and H Rappaport, Malignant lymphoma, lymphoblastic. Cancer 38:964-983, 1976

4. Jaffe, ES, EM Shevach, MM Frank, et al, Nodular lymphoma: Evidence for origin from follicular B lymphocytes. N Engl J Med 290:813-819, 1974

5. Leech, JH, AD Glick, JA Waldron, et al, Malignant lymphomas of follicular center cell origin in man. I. Immunologic studies. J Natl Cancer Inst 54:11-22, 1975

6. Aisenberg, AC and JC Long, Lymphocyte surface characteristics in malignant lymphoma. Am J Med 58:300-306, 1975

7. Chabner, BA, RE Johnson, VT DeVita, et al, Sequential staging in non-Hodgkin's lymphoma. Cancer Treat Rep 61:993-997, 1977

8. Qazi, R, AC Aisenberg and JC Long, The natural history of nodular lymphoma. Cancer 37:1923-1927, 1976

9. Mann, RB, ES Jaffe and CW Berard, Malignant lymphomas - A conceptual understanding of morphologic diversity. Am J Pathol 94:103-192, 1979.

10. Jones, EE, Z Fuks, M Bull, et al, Non-Hodgkin's lymphomas. IV Clinicopathologic correlation in 405 cases. Cancer 31:806-823, 1973

11. Lukes, RJ and RD Collins, Immunologic characterization of human malignant lymphomas. Cancer 34:1488-1503, 1974

12. Lennert, K, H Stein and E Kaiserling, Cytological and functional criteria for the classification of malignant lymphomata. Brit J Cancer 31 Supp II:29-43, 1975

13. Fu, SM, RJ Winchester, T Feizi, et al, Idiotypic specificity of surface immunoglobulin and the maturation of leukemic bone marrow derived lymphocytes. Proc Natl Acad Sci USA 71:4487-4490, 1974,

14. Tonder, O, PA Morse and LJ Humphrey, Similarities of Fc receptors in human malignant tissue and normal lymphoid tissue. J Immunol 113:1162-1169, 1974

15. Weiner, MD, C Bianco and V Nussenzweig, Enhanced binding of neuraminidase-treated sheep erythrocytes to human T lymphocytes. Blood 42:939-946, 1973

16. Craddock, CG, R Longmire and R McMillan, Lymphocytes and the immune response (second of two parts) N Engl J Med 285:378-384, 1971

17. O'Connell, CJ, Detection of lymphocyte rosettes in tissues. N Engl J Med 289:1312-1313, 1973

18. Sandilands, GP, K Gray, A Cooney, et al, Formation of auto-rosettes by peripheral blood lymphocytes. Clin Exp Immunol 22:493-501, 1975

19. Lohrman, HP and L Novikovs, Rosette formation between human T lymphocytes and unsensitized Rhesus monkey erythrocytes. Clin Immunol Immunopath 3:99-111, 1974

20. Braganza, CM, G Stathopoulous, AJS Davies, et al, Lymphocyte: erythrocyte (L.E.) rosettes as indicators of the heterogeneity of lymphocytes in a variety of mammalian species. Cell 4:103-106, 1975

21. Ptovin, C, JL Tarpley and P Chretein, Thymus-derived lymphocytes in patients with solid malignancies. Clin Immunol Immunopathol 3:476-481, 1975

22. Wybran, J, MC Carr and HH Fudenberg, The human rosette-forming cell as a marker of a population of thymus-derived cells. J Clin Invest 51:2537-2543, 1972.

23. Brayland, RC, ES Jaffe, JW Burbach, et al, Similarities of surface characteristics of neoplastic well-differentiated lymphocytes from solid tissues and from peripheral blood. Cancer Res 36:1619-1625, 1976

24. Aisenberg, AC, Malignant lymphoma. N Engl J Med 288:883-890, 1973

25. Fu, SM, N Chiorazzi, HG Kunkel, et al, Induction of in vitro differentiation and immunoglobulin synthesis of human leukemic B lymphocytes. J Exp Med 148:1570-1578, 1978

26. Braylan, RC, JC Long, ES Jaffe, et al, Lymphoid neoplasm obscured by concomitant extensive epitherlioid granulomas. Report of three cases with similar clinicopathologic features. Cancer 39:1146-1155, 1977

27. Kanba, K, ES Jaffe, RC Braylan, et al, Alkaline phosphatase positive malignant lymphomas: a subtype of B cell lymphomas. Am J Clin Pathol 68:535-542, 1977

28. Banks, PM, JC Arseneau, HR Gralnick, et al, American Burkitt's lymphoma: a clinicopathologic study of 30 cases. II. Pathologic correlations. Am J Med 58:322-329, 1975

29. Fialkow, PJ, E Klein, G Klein, et al, Immunoglobulin and glucose-6-phosphate dehydrogenase as markers of cellular origin in Burkitt's lymphoma. J Ecp Med 138:89, 1973

22

30. Mann, RB, ES Jaffe, RC Braylan, et al, Non-endemic Burkitt's lymphoma: a B cell tumor related to germinal centers. N Engl J Med 295:685-691, 1976

31. Edelson, RL, CH Kirkpatrick, EM Shevach, et al, Preferential cutaneous infiltration by neoplastic thymus-derived lymphocytes: Morphologic and functional studies. Ann Intern Med 80:685-692, 1974

32. Brouet, JC, G Flandrin and H Seligmann, Indications of the thymus derived nature of the proliferating cells in six patients with Sezary's syndrome. N Engl J Med. 289:341, 1973

33. Broder, S, RL Edelson, MA Lutzner, et al, The Sezary syndrome. A malignant proliferation of helper T cells. J Clin Invest 58:1297-1306, 1976

34. Smith, JL, CW Barker, GP Clein, et al, Characterization of malignant mediastinal lymphoid neoplasm (Sternberg sarcoma) as thymic in origin. Lancet i:74, 1973

35. Kaplan, J, R Mastrangelo and WD Peterson, Jr, Childhood lymphoblastic lymphoma, a cancer of thymus-derived lymphocytes. Cancer Res 34:521, 1974

36. Jaffe, ES, RC Braylan, MM Frank, et al, Heterogeneity of immunologic markers and surface morphology in childhood lymphoblastic lymphoma. Blood 48:213-222, 1976

37. Gatein, JG, EE Schneeberger and E Merler, Analysis of human thymocyte subpopulations using discontinuous gradients of albumin: Precursor lymphocytes in human thymus. Europ J Immunol 5:312-317, 1975

38. Kersey, JH, A Sabad, K Gajl-Peczalska, et al, Acute lymphoblastic leukemia cells with T (thymus-derived) lymphocyte markers. Science 182:1355, 1973

39. Sen, L and L Borella, Clinical importance of lymphoblasts with T markers in childhood acute leukemia. N Engl J Med 292:828, 1975

40. Donlon, JA and ES Jaffe, Terminal deoxynucleotidyl transferase activity in malignant lymphomas. N Engl J Med 297:461-464, 1977

41. Morris, MW and FR Davey, Immunologic and cytochemical properties of histiocytic and mixed histiocytic-lymphocytic lymphomas. Am J Clin Pathol 63:403-414, 1975

42. Brouet, JC, JL Preud ' homme, G Flandrin, et al, Brief communication: Membrane markers in "histiocytic" lymphomas (reticulum cell sarcomas). J Natl Cancer Inst 56:631-633, 1976

43. Fischer, R and R Schmalzl, Uber hemmbarkeit der esterase-aktivitat in blutmonocyten durch natriumfluorid. Klin Wschr 42:751, 1964

44. Preud ' homme, JL and M Seligmann, Surface bound immunoglobulins as a cell marker in human lymphoproliferative diseases. Blood 40:777-794, 1972

45. Brouet, J, J Preud ' homme and J Bernard, Blast cells with monoclonal surface immunoglobulin in two cases of acute blast crisis supervening in chronic lymphocytic leukemia. Brit Med J 4:23-24, 1974

46. Flandrin, G, and JC Flandrin, The Sezary cell: Cytologic, cytochemical and immunologic features. Mayo Clin Proc 49:575-583, 1974

47. Brouet, JC, G Flandrin, M Sasportes, et al, Chronic lymphocytic leukemia of T cell origin. Immunological and clinical evaluation in 11 patients. Lancet ii:890-893, 1975

48. Catovsky, D, J Galetto, A Okos, et al, Cytochemical profile of B and T leukaemic lymphocytes with special reference to acute lymphoblastic leukaemia. J Clin Path 27:767-771, 1974

49. Stein, H, N Petersen, G Gaedicke, et al, Lymphoblastic lymphoma of convoluted or acid phosphatase type - a tumor of T-precursor cells. Int J Cancer 17:292-295, 1976

50. Broder, S and TA Waldman, Helper activity by lymphocytes derived from patients with the Sezary syndrome. Blood 52:481-493, 1978

51. Fisher, RI, ES Jaffe, RC Braylan, et al, Immunoblastic lymphadenopathy: evolution into a malignant lymphoma with plasmacytoid features. Am J Med 61:553-559, 1976

52. Azar, HA, ES Jaffe, CW Berard, et al, Diffuse large cell lymphomas (Reticulum cell sarcomas) - Correlation of morphological features with functional markers. (submitted)

53. Bollum, FJ, TP Keneklis, JA Donlon, et al, Immunofluorescent assay for terminal deoxynucleotidyl transferase in leukemia and lymphoma. (abstract). XVII Congress of the International Society of Hematology. July 23-29, 1978, Paris, France

54. Jaffe, ES, TP Keneklis, JA Donlon, et al. (manuscript in preparation)

STAGING AND TREATMENT OF NON-HODGKIN'S LYMPHOMAS
Charles H. Diggs
Baltimore Cancer Research Program of the
Division of Cancer Treatment, National Cancer Institute
at the University of Maryland Hospital, Baltimore, Maryland

STAGING OF NON-HODGKIN'S LYMPHOMAS

Introduction

The non-Hodgkin's lymphomas are a somewhat heterogeneous group of diseases as can be seen from the previous article on their pathologic characteristics. Their clinical presentations may be similar to benign diseases, so before any treatment can be instituted for malignant lymphoma, two areas must be investigated. The first of these is biopsy of an area of clinical involvement to make the diagnosis, since few characteristics distinguish primary lymphoid malignancies from other benign disorders that cause lymphadenopathy. Secondly, the extent of disease (stage) must be adequately defined before appropriate therapy can be instituted.

In order to assist the accurate determination of stage, the physician must be familiar with the initial clinical manifestations of these diseases. A discussion of these presenting signs and symptoms is therefore in order.

Clinical Manifestations

Most patients with one of the non-Hodgkin's lymphomas present to the physician with painless, enlarged lymph nodes. The most common anatomic site of involvement is the cervical region, although somewhat in contrast to the sites of involvement with Hodgkin's disease, other lymph nodes are frequently involved. This lymphadenopathy usually is noted by the patient, although occasionally enlarged nodes may be found during a routine physical examination.

The presenting characteristic that most distinguishes these disorders from Hodgkin's disease is their predilection for involvement of sites other than lymph nodes, usually termed extranodal areas of disease. These sites may be the only areas evident at the onset--up to one-third of the time with some histologies--or more commonly are associated with wide-spread disease. Virtually any organ may be involved with lymphoma either as an isolated area or in conjunction with nodal disease. The most frequent of these is the gastrointestinal tract, with stomach involvement being the most common single site (1). Other extranodal areas include bone, skin, breast, testes, central nervous system, head and neck, or lung.

24

Some patients found to have a malignant lymphoma will present with constitutional or systemic symptoms as the only manifestation of disease or with both symptoms and lymphadenopathy. These include an unexplained fever of $38^{\circ}C$ or night sweats, or weight loss of greater than 10% of normal body weight. Approximately 10% of patients with a non-Hodgkin's lymphoma will have one or more of these symptoms at the time of diagnosis, and these patients have a poorer prognosis than those who are asymptomatic (2).

Because of the frequency of extranodal involvement with these disorders, initial evaluation of a patient who has been pathologically diagnosed must include attention to those areas most frequently infiltrated with lymphoma. These areas should be evaluated by the tests to be described but must include the bone marrow, liver, lung, kidney, central nervous system, and gastrointestinal tract. In addition, all lymph node-bearing areas must be examined for lymphomatous involvement. This process of total body evaluation is termed staging, either clinical, using physical exam, radionuclide and radiologic tests or pathologic using biopsies of areas frequently involved with lymphoma in addition to all clinical tests.

Staging Procedures

A staging system originally accepted for use for patients with Hodgkin's disease has been adapted for use with the non-Hodgkin's lymphomas. This system divides the stages by anatomic extent of disease and is described in table 1. This system has been modified by Peters (3) to include the frequent extranodal presentations seen with these disorders (table 2).

Unlike Hodgkin's disease, the non-Hodgkin's lymphomas tend to be widespread at the time of diagnosis. For this reason, the above mentioned staging systems may not be optimal for these disorders, although at present few alternatives exist. It is not inconceivable that a staging system could be designed distinctly for the non-Hodgkin's lymphomas incorporating response rates of various sites of disease or prognostic features as part of stage. For now, however, the Ann Arbor System, since its use has become widespread, should be used for therapeutic decisions.

Although it is true that most patients with non-Hodgkin's lymphomas have stage III or IV disease when first seen, it should not be assumed that all patients diagnosed will require chemotherapy for advanced disease. Patients with Hodgkin's disease must be proved to have advanced disease because most are early stage at the onset. The staging procedures for the non-Hodgkins lymphomas must be performed for the opposite reason: those with localized

Table 1
ANN ARBOR STAGING SYSTEM

Stage 1

Involvement of a single lymph node region (I) or of a single extralymphatic organ or site (I E)

Stage II

Involvement of two or more lymph node regions on the same side of the diaphragm (II) or localized involvement of an extralymphatic organ site and of one or more lymph node regions on the same side of the diaphragm (II E)

Stage III

Involvement of lymph node regions on both sides of the diaphragm (III) which may also be accompanied by localized involvement of an extralymphatic organ or site (III E) or by involvement of the spleen (III S) or both (III SE)

Stage IV

Diffuse or disseminated involvement of one or more extralymphatic organs or tissues with or without associated lymph node enlargement. Reasons for classifying the patient as Stage IV should be identified.

Table 2
PETERS MODIFICATION OF ANN ARBOR SYSTEM
FOR EXTRANODAL LYMPHOMAS

Stage I	Single extranodal site
Stage II	Single site + regional nodes
Stage III	One or two sites and lymph nodes beyond regional
Stage IV	Same as Ann Arbor

disease must be identified since therapeutically stage I or II disease would be amenable to radiotherapy. In addition, sites of disease should be identified to enable them to be followed for response to treatment. A list of procedures to be performed is seen in table 3.

Table 3

STAGING PROCEDURES

HISTORY AND PHYSICAL EXAMINATION

Chemistry

    Serum electrolytes

    Liver function tests

    Creatinine

    Serum protein electrophoresis

    Quantitative immunoglobulins

Hematology

    CBC

    Platelet count

    Differential white blood cell count

    Prothrombin time

    Coomb's test

Nuclear Medicine

    Liver-spleen scan

    Bone scan

    Gallium scan

Radiology

    Chest x-ray

    Whole lung tomography

    Upper G.I. series with small bowel
      follow-through

    Intravenous pyelogram

    Lymphangiogram

Miscellaneous

    Bone marrow biopsies

    Percutaneous liver biopsy

    Laparoscopy

    Laparotomy

    The most important staging procedure to be performed when a patient with known non-Hodgkin's lymphoma is first seen by a physician is the physical examination. This examination, together with the history obtained, will frequently reveal sites of nodal involvement that are widespread, making more invasive tests less important in determining treatment to be used. Special attention should be given to node bearing areas, especially those that may not frequently be examined, such as epitrochlear or submental sites. If, for instance, a patient first presents with cervical adenopathy, not only should the supradiaphragmatic node bearing areas be thoroughly examined but also the inguinal and femoral regions must be examined for nodes since, if nodes in these areas are found to contain lymphoma, chemotherapy should be employed since stage III disease would be documented. Nodal examination is also critical in those patients who present with extranodal areas of involvement. If nodal sites distant from the presenting site are involved, stage IV disease, not stage I_E, must be treated.

There are areas frequently involved by the non-Hodgkin's lymphomas that cannot be found by physical examination. Therefore, a thorough physical must be supplemented by several other procedures designed to find not only macroscopic evidence of lymphoma but also microscopic foci of disease that, if not detected and treated appropriately, would continue to grow and cause problems. These procedures generally fall into several categories: blood tests, radiologic and radionuclide studies, and pathologic examination of tissues. Each area will be discussed.

Blood Tests

Routine biochemical and hematologic tests need to be ordered prior to treatment as part of a thorough medical evaluation. Although few of these tests will by themselves affect any therapeutic decisions, baseline values are necessary and in fact may give clues to areas of disease involvement.

Serum electrolytes are rarely if ever affected by lymphoma, except if ureteral blockage is present causing renal dysfunction. An elevated serum creatinine will also be present with such blockage. Liver function tests may be abnormal but do not always indicate hepatic parenchymal lymphoma. These enzymes may be abnormal in the face of advanced disease not involving the liver, or may reflect extrahepatic biliary obstruction by enlarged porta hepatis nodes. Liver biopsy is the only sure way to document hepatic infiltration. The alkaline phosphatase may be elevated with advanced disease and may indicate liver or bone involvement. Abnormally high levels of uric acid may be found, especially in a rapidly growing lymphoma or in patients who have peripheral blood or bone marrow involvement. Patients with renal dysfunction also may have elevated uric acid levels. Serum protein levels usually are normal except in patients with far advanced disease, when a decreased serum albumin may be present.

Hematology tests may be more revealing than serum chemistries and may be great aids in determining stage of disease. A complete blood count may show selective or generalized abnormalities of the white cell, red cell, and platelet counts. White cells may be decreased, normal or increased in the presence of marrow lymphoma. The peripheral smear must be thoroughly examined for the presence of lymphoma regardless of the white blood cell count. Although one might expect leukopenia or a leukocytosis if marrow infiltration were present, frequently such infiltration may not be reflected in the peripheral blood counts. Anemia may be present with or without marrow lymphoma. Thrombocytopenia, however, usually is a strong indicator of marrow involvement.

RADIOLOGY AND NUCLEAR MEDICINE STUDIES

Once a complete history and physical examination have been obtained, and the patient has had appropriate blood studies, radiographs and isotopic scans should be obtained. A chest roentgenogram may show mediastinal widening, hilar or paratracheal adenopathy, or a parenchymal infiltrate or nodule. Infiltrates must not be assumed to be lymphoma in a febrile patient since many of these patients are prone to opportunistic infections because of immunodeficiencies.

If a plain chest radiograph does not show any abnormality, tomography of the mediastinum or whole-lung tomograms may be more sensitive at detecting lymphoma. Tomography is especially important in those patients who are thought to have limited stage or those who have infradiaphragmatic presentations with no supradiaphragmatic evidence of lymphoma.

An intravenous pyelogram (IVP) should be obtained in all patients. Its main use is in the detection of ureteral deviation or blockage by enlarged retroperitoneal nodes as seen in figure 1. An IVP, if abnormal, can also be used as a parameter by which to judge disease response since, if a good response to treatment is obtained, an abnormal IVP should become normal.   Upper

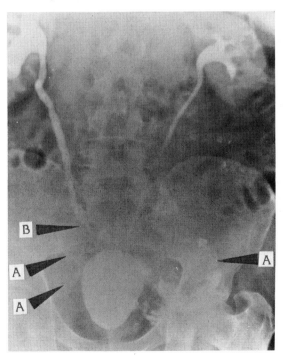

Figure 1: IVP in patient with non-Hodgkin's lymphoma. Note areas of enlarged nodes (A) outlined by lymphangiographic dye. One large node not easily seen (B) is producing ureteral constriction with hydronephrosis.

gastrointestinal radiographs may show bowel infiltration or, more frequently, indirect evidence of lymphoma by displacement or extrinsic compression of the bowel.

A bone survey is infrequently of use unless a patient has symptoms of bone pain. Not only is bony involvement infrequent in the non-Hodgkin's lymphomas, but also a bone survey is a relatively insensitive test in detecting this involvement.

A bipedal lymphangiogram should be obtained prior to therapy in every patient unless there is a major (pulmonary insufficiency) or relative (iodine sensitivity) contraindication. This procedure has been evaluated in several large series and is nearly 90% accurate when positive and equally predictive of the absence of abdominal lymphoma when negative (4). Inaccuracies of this procedure stem largely from its inability to evaluate mesenteric or nodes above the level of L-2, two areas frequently involved by non-Hodgkin's lymphomas. The

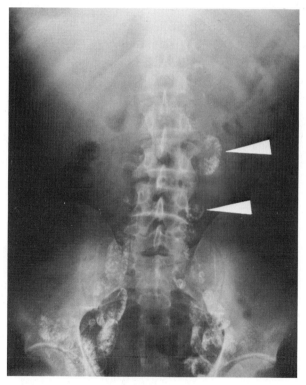

Figure 2: Large abdominal lymph nodes outlined by lymphangiogram. Of note nodes are large and have a speckled pattern with cut-out areas suggesting involvement with tumor.

lymphangiogram, in addition to its predictive capability is also useful to follow response to therapy since the nodes frequently retain dye for many months. Figures 1 and 2 show lymphangiograms which are positive for abdominal lymphoma.

SCANS

Radionuclide scans can be of use in the staging of lymphomas and should be performed for both staging and follow-up purposes. The liver-spleen scan is simple to perform, but its use is mainly limited to assessing organ size. Although many scans are performed in the hope of detecting parenchymal liver involvement or of finding indications of splenic lymphoma, rarely do the results of this scan affect therapy. This relative lack of usefulness is primarily due to the fact that in many instances of liver infiltration with non-Hodgkin's lymphoma, only microscopic foci of disease are discovered. The same is true for splenic involvement. The resolving power of present nuclear medicine techniques would not be expected to detect such involvement. Focal defects seen in the liver or the spleen, however, can indicate the presence of lymphoma.

Bone scans infrequently are helpful for staging due to the relatively infrequent bone involvement seen with these disorders. In fact, since many patients are in the older age groups, positive scans may only reflect osteoarthritis.

The radionuclide scan that is most helpful for staging the non-Hodgkin's lymphomas is the whole-body ^{67}gallium citrate scan, an example of which is seen in figure 3. Gallium is preferentially accumulated by inflammatory lesions and by certain malignancies. In general, the non-Hodgkin's lymphomas do accumulate gallium, but the degree of scan positivity is dependent on the degree of differentiation of the malignant cell. Several studies have examined gallium scans for staging and in general have found that less well-differentiated tumors accumulate gallium a greater percentage of the time than do well-differentiated lesions (5). Patients with histiocytic lymphomas, then, can be expected to have gallium uptake in sites of disease more often than do patients with well-differentiated lymphocytic lymphomas. The size of a lymphomatous lesion also affects gallium uptake with larger lesions being more frequently positive. Gallium scans do have drawbacks, however. Because gallium is secreted into the bowel, patients undergoing scans should have a thorough bowel preparation with cathartics and enemas, or scan positivity detected in the abdomen may be difficult to interpret. A gallium scan should be part of the initial staging evaluation both for delineating extent of disease at the onset and for establishing a baseline for whether the patient's tumor accumulates gallium. If the initial scan is negative even in the face of known areas of disease, further scans are of no use for assessing disease response.

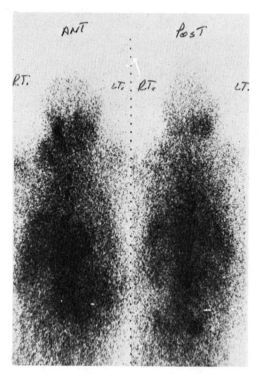

Figure 3: ^{67}Gallium scan showing increased uptake of radionuclide in cervical and inguinal areas corresponding to areas of palpable disease.

OTHER TESTS

Abdominal ultrasound and computerized axial tomography (CAT scan) are other procedures that help evaluate areas of potential disease involvement. Ultrasound can be useful in detecting enlarged retroperitoneal, porta hepatis, or mesenteric nodes but will not detect disease in normal-size nodes. The abdominal CAT scan, however, has the potential for finding areas of lymphoma undetected by other methods. Enlarged nodes not specified by lymphangiogram can be seen, including those in the high para-aortic and mesenteric areas. Microscopic foci of disease will not be detected. Studies of the use of abdominal CAT scans in the staging of lymphoma are underway. Thus the exact role of CAT scans remains to be established.

Pathologic Examinations

Not only should indirect evidence of lymphoma be sought by the use of the above tests but also biopsy evidence of sites known to be frequently involved should be sought. The sites of lymphoma that may not be detected prior to biopsy are bone marrow and liver.

Bone marrow infiltration is a frequent finding in the lymphocytic lymphomas and less frequent in the histiocytic varieties. All patients, regardless of histology, should have bilateral posterior iliac crest marrow biopsies, however. This is usually best accomplished by the use of a Jamshidi, Westerman-Jensen or similar needle which can be used to obtain both a marrow aspirate and biopsy with only one needle placement. Classically, lymphomatous infiltration of the marrow is in a focal paratrabecular pattern, but may be more widespread with large areas of marrow replaced by disease. Care must be taken to distinguish lymphoma from normal lymphoid follicles. Marrow involvement is always considered stage IV disease.

Liver infiltration should be sought since up to 30% of patients with lymphocytic histologies will have such involvement. This is detected by either percutaneous biopsy or with the use of peritoneoscopy, directing biopsies to areas that are suspicious, or taking random biopsies. Liver biopsy should however be reserved for those patients who have not been shown to have stage IV disease before biopsy.

Final Impact of Staging

Staging of the non-Hodgkin's lymphomas should proceed in the sequence outlined above. By the time all of the above tests have been completed, the vast majority of patients with non-Hodgkin's lymphomas will have been found to have stage III or IV disease, requiring chemotherapy. These patients will require no further staging evaluation. It is also important to remember that clinical stage at presentation may not be an accurate reflection of pathologic stage which frequently is advanced by the finding of small foci of disease not easily detected by clinical means. For those few patients who appear to have localized disease, staging laparotomy should be employed to document that the disease is indeed localized. This laparotomy should employ all of the procedures used in the evaluation of patients with Hodgkin's disease as outlined in table 4. Special attention should be directed to the mesenteric nodes since these nodes are frequently involved in the non-Hodgkin's lymphomas. When adequate pathologic stage is assessed, the patient is ready for treatment.

Table 4

PROCEDURES AT STAGING LAPAROTOMY

Splenectomy

Liver Biopsies
    Wedge biopsy
    Needle biopsy right and left
     lobes
    Suspicious lesions

Lymph Node Biopsies
    Splenic hilum
    Porta hepatis
    Mesenteric
    Bilateral para-aortic
    Bilateral iliac

Iliac Crest Bone Marrow Biopsy

Other as Indicated
    Biopsy of bone lesions
    Peripheral lymph node biopsies

TREATMENT OF NON-HODGKIN'S LYMPHOMAS

General

The majority of patients with one of the malignant lymphomas of the non-Hodgkin's type will respond to appropriate therapy, often with complete resolution of their disease. This statement is becoming increasingly true as newer methods of treatment are developed, but it has not always been so recognized. Successful therapy has in general lagged behind the spectacular success that has been achieved in the last decade in the treatment of Hodgkin's disease. Reasons for this slower rate of achievement are several and include the lack of appropriate studies to determine the extent of disease at the time of an extranodal presentation; the relative resistance of some types of non-Hodgkin's lymphomas to megavoltage radiation therapy; and the slow realization that these disorders are, in the vast majority of instances, truly systemic diseases at the time of their clinical detection. Overall, even considering the relative lack of major breakthroughs in therapy, the patient who is diagnosed as having a non-Hodgkin's lymphoma has a better chance now of having long-term control of his disease than he would have had even 10 years ago. As will be discussed, some of these patients have a very real chance of being cured with present day treatment modalities.

As with many neoplastic diseases, three modalities of therapy are available for the treatment of the non-Hodgkin's lymphomas: surgery, radiotherapy, and chemotherapy. Each of these has its place in management, but whether it is used alone or they are used in combination primarily depends on the extent or stage of the lymphoma. Most patients with one of these lymphoid malignancies will be found to have disseminated, systemic disease at the completion of the staging evaluation. These patients are usually most appropriately treated with chemotherapy. There remains a small proportion of patients, however, who even after all studies including staging laparotomy have been done, will be found to have relatively local disease (stage I or II). It is with these few patients that surgery and radiotherapy are the most useful. Since surgery, irradiation, and chemotherapy all can be used therapeutically for the non-Hodgkin's lymphomas, each will be discussed separately.

Surgery

The greatest contribution of surgery to the treatment of these disorders is in the performance of the diagnostic biopsy. Since many patients come to the medical oncologist having already been diagnosed, the importance of this diagnostic function is frequently overlooked. A peripheral node is the most frequent site of biopsy, and should cause little diagnostic trouble since the node is usually excised in toto and an adequate sample of tissue is obtained for pathologic diagnosis. Even if confusion over the proper diagnosis arises, these nodes are usually large enough that tissue is available for further sections and additional stains. Rarely is a frozen section indicated in a peripheral node biopsy, and if one is performed care must be taken not to freeze the entire specimen since freezing may destroy critical cellular characteristics and make interpretation difficult.

Another mode of presentation of these disorders may be with abdominal signs, either with an abdominal mass or with gastrointestinal involvement. A surgeon usually makes the diagnosis of abdominal lymphoma since many of these patients may not have peripheral adenopathy and require exploratory laparotomy. In these instances, especially when the diagnosis of lymphoma is being considered, the opportunity to do a thorough staging laparotomy should be taken rather than doing only a biopsy of the abnormal area. All too frequently, such patients do not have disease outside the abdomen, leaving their true stage in doubt if node biopsies, liver biopsies, and splenectomy have not been done at the time of the initial surgery. These patients may then need further surgery if an inadequate first procedure has been done.

Surgery may be truly therapeutic, rather than diagnostic, in occasional patients with non-Hodgkin's lymphoma. This situation may occur in those patients who present with an extranodal site of disease which can be totally excised. Any organ may be the presenting site of a malignant lymphoma. The most frequent extranodal presenting site is the gastrointestinal tract, with the stomach being the most frequent area of involvement. The literature concerning the surgical removal of these sites of disease suggests that a certain percentage - in some series up to one-half of these patients - may be cured by the surgical procedure itself. Most of these series, however, fail to adequately stage the patients. When staging is performed in patients with extranodal presentations, the vast majority can be found to have disseminated disease (6-8). Obviously these patients could not be cured by any local surgical procedure. If these patients are adequately staged and if this staging evaluation (including a staging laparotomy) does not find evidence of further sites of lymphomatous involvement, it is conceivable that adequate surgical removal of an extranodal primary lymphoma may be curative.

Radiotherapy

Megavoltage radiation therapy will cause regression of nearly all areas of non-Hodgkin's lymphoma that are irradiated. This therapeutic use of irradiation has been known for many years but in most series radiotherapy has not been as curative as it has been for Hodgkin's disease. Two reasons for this relative lack of success are now evident. Most importantly, adequate staging has only recently been recognized as being critical for making correct therapeutic decisions. One cannot hope to control what in most cases is a systemic disease with local therapy. Secondly, the local recurrence in an irradiated field varies with the histologic subtype of lymphoma.

At Stanford, a study by Fuks and Kaplan (9) demonstrated that local recurrence is dependent on cell type with poorly differentiated lymphocytic and mixed lymphomas, whether in a nodular or a diffuse pattern, having fewer recurrences as the dose of radiotherapy approached 4000 rads. Diffuse histiocytic lymphomas, however, did not show this dose response, with more recurrences at 5500 rads than were seen at 2000 rads. This study corroborated what is frequently seen in the clinic after radiotherapy for control of these disorders. Sites involved with lymphocytic lymphoma are well controlled, but the patient may suffer the consequences of distant spread, whereas sites of histiocytic lymphoma frequently re-grow after irradiation and local manifestations of the disease are a prominent feature. Airway, ureteral, or gastrointestinal obstruction by diffuse histiocytic lymphoma may initially be relieved by radiation therapy, only to recur and, because of potential radiation damage to normal tissues, not be amenable to further irradiation.

Knowing the responses of the lymphomas to irradiation, several studies have utilized radiotherapy for patients with these disorders. Response rates have been excellent with nearly all patients treated having complete regressions of their diseases. The relapse rates following the achievement of a complete remission have been relatively high, however, with only about one-half of the patients achieving long-term control of their diseases. Relapse rates have been somewhat dependent on the clinical stage of the disease at the time of irradiation with stage I patients relapsing from 40 to 75% of the time if a nodular lymphoma were treated, and 40 to 100% if a diffuse histology were present (10-13). Stage II patients have fared less well, with stage III lymphomas doing better (14) or about the same (15) as stage II (table 5).

Table 5

PERCENT RELAPSE AFTER RADIOTHERAPY

Investigator	Stage	Percent Relapse Nodular		Diffuse
Hellman (10)	I	40		100
	I & II		50	
Reddy (11)	I	44		45
	II	46		80
Cox (14)	III	35		--
Bush (12)	I & II		55	
Jones (13)				
PDL + MIXED	I	75		40
	II	75		100
Histiocytic	I	0		55
	II	70		75
Glatstein (15)	III	67		80

These results with radiotherapy must be analyzed further, however, in order to get a true picture of the effectiveness of irradiation. First of all, most of the studies outlined in table 5 have not used aggressive staging procedures. The patients, therefore, are clinically staged as opposed to being pathologically or surgically staged. Most patients in these series underwent lymphangiograms and bone marrow aspirates, but few had marrow biopsies, liver biopsies, or staging laparotomies. The relapse percentages may therefore be high because of occult foci of disease that received no therapy and would be expected to become clinically manifest in due time. Thus "relapse" after radiotherapy may not represent escape of the disease from treatment, but may be only a manifestation of initial undertreatment. The study that appears to come closest to accurate staging is that of Cox (14) who delivered radiotherapy of curative intent to patients with stage III nodular disease with excellent results. At the time of publication, 10 of 22 patients treated had relapsed, but 3 of those who relapsed were made disease free with further radiotherapy. A similar group of patients treated at Stanford (15), however, fared less well, with 67% of those with nodular disease relapsing. In the Stanford study, the follow-up period was nearly twice as long.

A second criticism of these studies of radiotherapy is that not all of them specify where the disease recurred. It is of importance to document whether the disease became evident in previously irradiated sites (true recurrence) or in previously untreated areas (relapse). The former would suggest biologic resistance whereas the latter would mean inadequate evaluation of the initial extent of disease. Lastly, it might be expected that very few patients with truly localized lymphoma actually exist since 90% are systemic from the time of diagnosis. These patients may be curable by radiotherapy so it is exceedingly important to identify them.

Adjuvant Chemotherapy. Hopefully it is clear from the preceding discussion that the role of radiation therapy as a curative modality of treatment for the non-Hodgkin's lymphomas is as yet unsettled. Because of the high recurrence/relapse rate of patients treated with radiotherapy alone, studies of adjuvant chemotherapy (see below) have been performed in attempts to prolong the disease-free interval. It is now clear that this type of therapy significantly prolongs remission duration for patients with early stage Hodgkin's disease and significantly prolongs survival in subsets of these patients over those treated only with irradiation. In two large series of patients with non-Hodgkin's treated with either radiotherapy alone or radiotherapy followed by combination chemotherapy, results have been conflicting, with one study (16) showing an advantage for those treated with combined modality therapy in disease-free interval but not in overall survival. This advantage was seen primarily in patients with diffuse lymphomas, and because most (70%) of the patients treated had a diffuse histology, this advantage was seen for the entire group. Survival at 3 years was not significantly different with the addition of chemotherapy; aggressive post-relapse treatment was credited with prolonging the survival of the relapsers. Another study of adjuvant chemotherapy (17), however, failed to find significant differences between the two treatment groups. No subset of patients by stage or histology benefitted by the addition of chemotherapy following radiotherapy.

From these two studies it is difficult to accurately assess whether or not adjuvant chemotherapy is beneficial for patients with early stage non-Hodgkin's lymphomas. Once again, the previous comments about accurate staging must apply, since presumably only clinical staging was done in these studies. The answer to whether or not chemotherapy should be given after radiotherapy in this patient group will have to await further studies of adequately staged patients.

Total Body Irradiation. One other method of delivering radiotherapy to patients with non-Hodgkin's lymphomas is total body irradiation (TBI) (18-22). This method, as its name implies, does not direct the radiotherapy beam to only lymph node bearing areas, but rather delivers relatively low dose (100-500 rads) irradiation to the entire patient. Usually, half of the patient is treated on a daily to weekly basis, delivering 10-20 rads to alternate halves of the body. The treatment is generally well tolerated with thrombocytopenia being the pre-dominant dose limiting factor. Complete remissions have been achieved, primarily in patients with lymphocytic histologies. Compared to combination chemotherapy, TBI has been equally effective (23). Although many studies (table 6) have been performed to assess the efficacy of TBI, most have been pilot studies and the results have varied. The role of total body irradiation in the treatment of patients with non-Hodgkin's lymphomas is not yet established.

Table 6

TOTAL BODY IRRADIATION

Author	Schedule	Total Dose (Rads)	Complete Response (%)
Chaffey (18)	15 rads 2x/week	150	80
Qasim (19)	10 rads 3x/week	100-300	75
Johnson (20)	10 rads daily	100-150	69
Brace (21)	15 rads weekly	85-196	29
Garrett (22)	10-50 rads daily	125-500	29

Chemotherapy

As has been mentioned, nearly all patients having one of these disorders will have extensive disease when first seen. When staging is completed, some patients will have stage I or II disease; these patients will be candidates for radiotherapy alone or in combination with chemotherapy (see above). The remainder will require systemic therapy since they have systemic disease. This therapy will usually mean treatment with chemotherapy.

There are a number of chemotherapeutic agents that are available for use for the non-Hodgkin's lymphomas (table 7). Agents that have had the most extensive use are the alkylating agents, vinca alkaloids, and corticosteroids. Drugs from each of these groups have been studied for use as single agents, and the alkylating agents have been the most studied.

Table 7
CHEMOTHERAPEUTIC AGENTS FOR LYMPHOMA

Alkylating Agents
    Nitrogen Mustard
    Cyclophosphamide
    Chlorambucil

Vinca Alkaloids
    Vincristine
    Vinblastine

Corticosteroids
    Prednisone

Antibiotics
    Adriamycin
    Bleomycin

Nitrosoureas
    CCNU
    BCNU
    Streptozotocin

Antimetabolites
    Methotrexate

Miscellaneous
    Procarbazine
    VM-26
    DTIC

Several reports have shown that alkylating agents alone can be effective treatment for non-Hodgkin's lymphomas. Early studies suggested that chlorambucil (24) or cyclophosphamide (25) have clinical utility in these patients but these reports were published prior to the widespread use of the Rappaport classification system. Hence activity reported in "lymphosarcoma" or "reticulum cell sarcoma", is of limited value because of the lack of precise histologic correlation. Jones (26) in a retrospective review of 110 patients with these disorders classified by the Rappaport method reported response rates to either cyclophosphamide or chlorambucil that were dependent on the histologic subtype. Nodular lymphomas responded with greater frequency than did diffuse histologies and among the nodular types, poorly differentiated lymphocytic (NPDL) was the most responsive. Forty-eight percent of the patients with NPDL histology were able to achieve a complete remission, but only 5 percent of those with diffuse histiocytic lymphomas (DHL) were able to do so. It is likely, however, that these response rates are somewhat inflated since aggressive restaging procedures were not used to document remission status. High-dose cyclophosphamide (27) (1500 mg/m^2 every 3 to 4 weeks) has also been reported as effective therapy for nodular lymphomas. Forty-two percent of the patients with nodular histologies achieved a complete remission, but none of the patients with diffuse histologies completely responded.

Table 8

COMBINATION CHEMOTHERAPY FOR LYMPHOMA

Drugs	Reference	Complete Remission (%)	
		Nodular	Diffuse
Cyclophosphamide Vincristine Prednisone (COP)	Bagley (28)	61	43
COP	Lenhard (29)	50	43
Adriamycin Vincristine Prednisone (HOP)	McKelvey (31)	67	60
Cyclophosphamide + HOP (CHOP)	McKelvey (31)	78	67
COP + Procarbazine (COPP)	Stein (32)	62	50
CHOP + Bleomycin	Rodriguez (34)	63	68
Adriamycin Bleomycin Prednisone	Monfardini (36)	80	44
Bleomycin Adriamycin + COP (BACOP)	Schein (35)	--	48
Methotrexate Cyclophosphamide Vincristine	Lauria (37)	57	78

Single agents have also been combined and in general, the results obtained with these combinations have been superior to those obtained with single drugs (table 8). The most widely used of these combinations has been COP or CVP which groups cyclophosphamide, vincristine, and prednisone. Although these three drugs have been used together frequently, the dosage and schedules have varied so that COP or CVP does not have the same meaning in all centers. Cyclophosphamide has been given daily orally (28), weekly (29), or on a high-dose intermittent schedule (30). Comparisons between these studies are difficult since methods of staging, make-up of the patient population, and thoroughness of re-staging differ among them, but in general, results appear equivalent with all schedules. Complete remission rates with the 3-drug combination have been generally near 50%, with nodular lymphomas responding more frequently than diffuse histologies.

Several agents have been substituted in or added to CVP in attempts to improve the complete response rates. Adriamycin (hydroxyl-daunomycin) has been substituted for cyclophosphamide (HOP) with a slight increase in response rate (31). The addition of Adriamycin (CHOP) further increases the complete remission percentage both in nodular and diffuse lymphomas (31). Procarbazine (32) has been added with little improvement in response rates and the addition of BCNU likewise appears to confer no benefit (33). Nitrogen mustard and procarbazine with vincristine and prednisone (MOPP) appears equivalent to CVP (30). Bleomycin added to CHOP (34) adds no more activity than is seen with CHOP alone, although appears to be of benefit in patients with histiocytic lymphoma when used in a different schedule (35). Other regimens not employing the nucleus of CVP have also been reported with good results. Adriamycin, bleomycin and prednisone is an effective combination (36), as is methotrexate, cyclophosphamide and vincristine (MEV) (37).

Nearly all investigators would agree on the necessity of combination chemotherapy for patients with histologic subtypes that are considered to have poorer prognoses. Most of these less favorable histologies are of diffuse architecture, either poorly differentiated lymphocytic (DPDL), mixed lympho-cytic/histiocytic (DM), or histiocytic lymphoma (DHL). Although patients with these types of lymphomas respond less frequently to chemotherapy than do "favorable" ones (diffuse well differentiated lymphocytic - DWDL, NPDL, or nodular mixed - NM) there exists a subpopulation of these who have a reasonable chance of long-term disease-free survival. Aggressive therapy directed toward this possibility would then seem worthwhile. Less clear is what is the best therapeutic course for patients with the less aggressive, more indolent type of lymphoma - DWDL, NPDL, or NM. Suggestions for approaching this group of patients have ranged from no initial treatment, withholding any therapy until symptoms of bulky nodes or life-threatening organ involvement intervene; to single agent chemotherapy; to combination chemotherapy. Which of these methods of managing these patients is of the most benefit is a widely debated issue, and arguments supporting each view can be found (38,39).

Portlock and Rosenberg (40) have suggested a "wait and see" approach for patients with favorable histologies. Patients whose diseases are asymptomatic do not have bulky adenopathy, or do not have life-threatening complications are followed without treatment until symptoms requiring therapy appear as they will in the majority of patients. The survival curves reported for a highly selected group of patients treated in this manner were relatively good, reflecting in part the indolent nature of their diseases, and did not differ significantly from the survival curve generated for a group of patients on a randomized treatment protocol. What the exact criteria were for choosing patients to be followed untreated are not clear. Also not answered by this study is whether or not these patients may have done even better or even "cured" had they been treated from the time of diagnosis. One can only say that there exists a group of patients with these disorders who may not require immediate treatment.

Single agent chemotherapy has been compared to combinations of drugs in 3 studies (38,41,42) and in each case, combination chemotherapy has given a higher number of complete remissions. Whether or not it is important to attain a complete remission, since remissions are not durable and long-term control of nodular lymphomas is infrequent, is a question that also is debated. Some studies (43) show no significant survival differences among those who respond fully, partially or not at all, while we (39) have shown highly significant differences, with complete responders living longer than non-responders. If it be true that the attainment of a complete remission significantly prolongs survival for patients with nodular lymphoma, then therapy should be designed to achieve high complete response rates. Since combinations are superior to single agents in this capacity, it would seem prudent to try combination chemotherapy as initial treatment. Randomized trials of no initial treatment, single agent therapy, and combination chemotherapy in unselected patients may need to be performed to help answer this question.

Re-staging. Whatever therapy is employed for the treatment of the non-Hodgkin's lymphomas, it is important to accurately assess not only initial stage of the disease, but also the response to therapy. Therefore, when a patient is thought to have achieved a clinical complete remission, tests that were performed prior to treatment should be repeated. Only those tests that showed evidence of lymphoma need to be re-done, i.e. if a scan, radiograph, or biopsy was initially negative, it need not be repeated. If further studies show continued presence of lymphoma, treatment should be continued for 2 to 3 more cycles and the tests done again. Persistent disease at that point requires a change of therapy. Care must be exercised in interpretation of these repeated tests, however, since false positive results can occur, especially with the interpretation of repeat lymphangiograms. In our experience, fully 75% of those nodes read as positive on repeat studies proved negative at laparotomy.

Maintenance. Whether or not maintenance therapy is indicated for these patients after a pathologically documented complete remission is attained is an unstudied question. Studies of maintenance have been reported, but these were in the era prior to the use of the Rappaport histologic classification system, so are difficult to interpret. Since nodular lymphomas tend to relapse with time but remissions in patients with diffuse lymphomas, especially those with DHL, seem to be durable, perhaps maintenance treatment may be appropriate for certain histologies. Obviously further studies in this area are needed.

Conclusions and Recommendations

The strongest determinant of how patients with one of the non-Hodgkin's malignant lymphomas should be treated is the pathologic stage of the disease. Stage can only be accurately determined by a thorough evaluation of all sites likely to be involved with lymphoma. Only when this staging has been completed can therapy begin. Treatment should be approached as follows:

Stage I & II Any histology. Radiotherapy to at least one node bearing area beyond what is known to be involved should be given to a dose of 4000 rads. Abdominal ports should encompass mesenteric nodes if they are known to be involved. Otherwise, ports analogous to those used for Hodgkin's disease are appropriate. Chemotherapy as adjuvant following irradiation is currently optional.

Stage IE Any histology. Surgical removal if possible may be curative. Radiotherapy alone without surgery may offer good control. Radiotherapy after surgery is optional.

Stage III or IV DPDL, DM, DHL, NH. Combination chemotherapy with three, four, or five drug regimens will give a high percentage of complete remissions that may be of long duration. Patients who fail to achieve a complete remission should be treated with a different combination of drugs.

Stage III or IV DWDL; NPDL, NM. Various options for treatment are available.   If the disease appears stable, treatment may be withheld until symptoms appear. Single agent therapy or combination chemotherapy may be used, with more patients on combinations achieving complete remission. Total body irradiation appears useful but is currently investigational.

Treatment of these disorders has shown marked improvement within the last 10 years so that the majority of patients will have responses and many will have long-term control of their disease and prolonged survival. Further progress toward cure will depend on the development of newer agents and upon newer combinations which have even greater activity for patients with the non-Hodgkin's lymphomas.

REFERENCES

1. Freeman, C, JW Berg, and SJ Cutler, Occurrence and prognosis of extranodal lymphomas. Cancer 29:252-260, 1972

2. Bloomfield, CD, A Goldman, F Dick, et al, Multivariate analysis of prognostic factors in the non-Hodgkin's malignant lymphomas. Cancer 33:870-879, 1974

3. Peters, MV, RS Bush, TC Brown, et al, The place of radiotherapy in the control of non-Hodgkin's lymphomata. Br J Cancer 31(II):386-401, 1975

4. Goffinet DR, R Warnke, NR Dunnick, et al, CLinical and surgical (laparotomy) evaluation of patients with non-Hodgkin's lymphomas. Cancer Treat Rep 61:981-992, 1977

5. Levi, JA, MJ O'Connell, WL Murphy, et al, Role of [67]gallium citrate scanning in the management of non-Hodgkin's lymphoma. Cancer 36:1690-1741, 1975

6. Long, JC, MC Mihm, and R Qazi, Malignant lymphoma of the skin. Cancer 38:1282-1296, 1976

7. Reimer, RR, BA Chabner, RC Young, et al, Lymphoma presenting in bone. Ann Intern Med 87:50-55, 1977

8. Woolley, PV, CK Osborne, JA Levi, et al, Extranodal presentation of non-Hodgkin's lymphomas in the testis. Cancer 38:1026-1035, 1976

9. Fuks, Z and HS Kaplan, Recurrence rates following radiation therapy of nodular and diffuse malignant lymphomas. Radiology 108:675-684, 1973

10. Hellman, S, JT Chaffey, DS Rosenthal, et al, The place of radiation therapy in the treatment of non-Hodgkin's lymphomas. Cancer 39:843-851, 1977

11. Reddy, S, VS Saxena, EV Pellettiere, et al, Early nodal and extra-nodal non-Hodgkin's lymphomas. Cancer 40:98-104, 1977

12. Bush, RS, M Gospodarowicz, J Sturgeon, et al, Radiation therapy of localized non-Hodgkin's lymphoma. Cancer Treat Rep 61:1129-1136, 1977

13. Jones, SE, Z Fuks, HS Kaplan, et al, Non-Hodgkin's lymphomas: V. Results of radiotherapy. Cancer 32:682-691, 1973

14. Cox, JD, Central lymphatic irradiation to low dose for advanced nodular lymphoreticular tumors (non-Hodgkin's lymphoma). Radiology 126:767-772, 1978

15. Glatstein, E, Z Fuks, DR Goffinet, et al, Non-Hodgkin's lymphomas of stage III extent. Cancer 37:2806-2812, 1976

48

16. Lattuada, A, G Bonadonna, F Milani, et al, Adjuvant chemotherapy with CVP after radiotherapy (RT) in stage I-II non-Hodgkin's lymphomas. In Adjuvant Therapy of Cancer, Salmon SE and SE Jones (eds). Amsterdam, Elsevier/North Holland Biomedical Press, 1977, p 537-544

17. Panahon, A, JH Kaufman, JA Grasso, et al, Randomized study of radiation therapy (RT) vs RT and chemotherapy (CT) on stage IA-IIIB non-Hodgkin's lymphoma (NHL). Proc Am Soc Clin Oncol 18:321, 1977

18. Chaffey, JT, S Hellman, DS Rosenthal, et al, Total-body irradiation in the treatment of lymphocytic lymphoma. Cancer Treat Rep 61:1149-1152, 1977

19. Qasim, MM, Total body irradiation in non-Hodgkin lymphoma. Strahlentherapie 149:364-367, 1975

20. Johnson, RE, Total body irradiation (TBI) as primary therapy for advanced lymphosarcoma. Cancer 35:242-246, 1975

21. Brace, K, MJ O'Connell, V Vogel, et al, Total body radiation therapy for disseminated lymphosarcoma: results of a pilot study. Cancer Chemother Rep 58:401-405, 1974

22. Garrett, MJ and S Das, A preliminary study in treatment of non-Hodgkin's lymphoma by whole body irradiation. Clin Radiol 27:409-414, 1976

23. Young, RC, RE Johnson, GP Canellos, et al, Advanced lymphocytic lymphoma: randomized comparisons of chemotherapy and radiotherapy, alone or in combination. Cancer Treat Rep 61:1153-1159, 1977

24. Galton, DAG, LG Israels, JDN Nabarro, et al, Clinical trials of p-(DI-2-chloroethylamino)-phenyl-butyric acid (CB 1348) in malignant lymphoma. Brit Med J 2:1172-1176, 1955

25. Carbone, PP and C Spurr, Management of patients with malignant lymphoma: A comparative study with cyclophosphamide and vinca alkaloids. Cancer Res 28:811-822, 1968

26. Jones, SE, SA Rosenberg, HS Kaplan, et al, Non-Hodgkin's lymphomas II: Single agent chemotherapy. Cancer 30:31-38, 1972

27. O'Connell, MJ, PH Wiernik and JC Sutherland, Highdose intermittent intravenous cyclophosphamide in non-Hodgkin's lymphomas: longterm patient follow up. Oncology 33:170-172, 1976

28. Bagley, CM, VT DeVita Jr, CW Berard, et al, Advanced lymphosarcoma: intensive cyclical combination chemotherapy with cyclophosphamide, vincristine, and prednisone. Ann Intern Med 76:227-234, 1972

29. Lenhard, RE Jr, RL Prentice, AH Owens Jr, et al, Combination chemotherapy of the malignant lymphomas. Cancer 38:1052-1059, 1976

30. Benjamin, RS, PH Wiernik, MJ O'Connell, et al, A comparison of cyclophosphamide, vincristine, and prednisone (COP) with nitrogen mustard, vincristine, procarbazine, and prednisone (MOPP) in the treatment of nodular, poorly differentiated lymphocytic lymphoma. Cancer 38:1896-1902, 1976

31. McKelvey, EM, JA Gottlieb, HE Wilson, et al, Hydroxyldaunomycin (Adriamycin) combination chemotherapy in malignant lymphoma. Cancer 38:1484-1493, 1976

32. Stein, RS, EM Moran, RK Desser, et al, Combination chemotherapy of lymphomas other than Hodgkin's disease. Ann Intern Med 81:601-609, 1974

33. Durant, JR, RA Gams, AA Bartolucci, et al, BCNU with and without cyclophosphamide, vincristine, and prednisone (COP) and cycle-active therapy in non-Hodgkin's lymphoma. Cancer Treat Rep 61:1085-1096, 1977

34. Rodriguez, V, F Cabanillas, MA Burgess, et al, Combination chemotherapy ("CHOP-Bleo") in advanced (non-Hodgkin) malignant lymphoma. Blood 49:325-333, 1977

35. Schein, PS, VT DeVita Jr, S Hubbard, et al, Bleomycin, Adriamycin, cyclophosphamide, vincristine and prednisone (BACOP) combination chemotherapy in the treatment of diffuse histiocytic lymphoma. Annals Intern Med 85:417-422, 1976

36. Monfardini, S, G Tancini, M DeLena, et al, Cyclophosphamide, vincristine and prednisone (CVP) versus Adriamycin, bleomycin, and prednisone (ABP) in stage IV non-Hodgkin's lymphomas. Med Ped Oncol 3:67-74, 1977

37. Lauria, F, M Baccarani, M Fiacchini, et al, Methotrexate, cyclophosphamide and vincristine (MEV regimen) for non-Hodgkin's lymphoma. Europ J Cancer 11:343-349, 1975

38. Portlock, CS and SA Rosenberg, Chemotherapy of the non-Hodgkin's lymphomas: the Stanford experience. Cancer Treat Rep 61:1049-1055, 1977

39. Diggs, CH and PH Wiernik, Nodular lymphoma - complete remission prolongs survival. Blood 52 (Suppl 1):246, 1978

40. Portlock CS and SA Rosenberg, No initial therapy for stage III and IV non-Hodgkin's lymphomas of favorable histologic types. Ann Intern Med 90:10-13, 1979

41. Kennedy BJ, CD Bloomfield, DT Kiang, et al, Combination versus successive single agent chemotherapy in lymphocytic lymphoma. Cancer 41:23-28, 1978

42. Lister, TA, MH Cullen, MEJ Beard, et al, Comparison of combined and single agent chemotherapy in non-Hodgkin's lymphoma of favourable histological type. Brit Med J 1:533-537, 1978

43. Ezdinli, EZ, W Costello, RE Lenhard Jr, et al, Survival of nodular versus diffuse pattern lymphocytic poorly differentiated lymphoma. Cancer 41:1990-1996, 1978

CURRENT ISSUES IN THE MANAGEMENT OF PATIENTS WITH HODGKIN'S DISEASE

Peter H. Wiernik

Baltimore Cancer Research Program of the
Division of Cancer Treatment, National Cancer Institute
at the University of Maryland Hospital, Baltimore, Maryland

INTRODUCTION

There is currently great and often heated debate over some important aspects of the management of patients with Hodgkin's disease. New data concerning the proper staging of patients have been developed at several centers, but these data and their implications for staging and management have not been universally accepted. Research at several institutions has indicated that a combined modality approach to some patients with early stage disease offers the best chance of prolonged disease free survival. However, some investigators have argued that overall survival is not enhanced by such aggressive treatment because "salvage" chemotherapy will cure a significant fraction of radiation failures. "Salvage" therapy, however, has not been so effective in all studies. Those who favor the radiotherapy alone approach to all patients with early stage disease argue additionally that the frequency of second malignancies in patients with Hodgkin's disease is greatest in patients who receive intensive combined modality therapy. Others point out that, while this may be true, closer examination of relevant data demonstrates that the incidence of second malignancies is greatest in patients who receive intensive radiotherapy initially, relapse, and then receive intensive combination chemotherapy as reinduction treatment. It must be noted that such reinduction chemotherapy constitutes "salvage" therapy.

Recently, some early data have demonstrated the potential of combination chemotherapy alone for successful induction of complete remission in early Hodgkin's disease. Although such therapy may be associated with more acute toxicity than radiotherapy, the long term permanent complications of radiotherapy may be greater. More remission duration data must be developed, however, before combination chemotherapy can be recommended as an alternative to radiotherapy for early stage disease.

The purpose of this paper is to discuss some of these issues critically and to make new recommendations based on the data for the management of patients with Hodgkin's disease.

51

COMBINED MODALITY APPROACH TO HODGKIN'S DISEASE
PRIMARILY CONFINED TO LYMPH NODES

The results of two major studies comparing radiotherapy alone to radiotherapy followed by chemotherapy for early stage Hodgkin's disease have shown a statistically significant improvement in remission duration after combined modality treatment (1,2). In both studies, overall survival is also better in the combined modality group compared to the radiotherapy group but the differences are not significant in the Stanford study (1). The lack of a statistically significant difference in overall survival has led some to recommend radiotherapy alone for patients with early stage Hodgkin's disease. They prefer to withhold combination chemotherapy until the patient relapses. This approach is justified by three observations. First, this approach will spare a majority of patients chemotherapy, since a majority of patients remain disease free after radiotherapy alone. Secondly, post relapse "salvage" chemotherapy is said to be highly successful (3) - so successful, in fact, that the ultimate survival of groups of patients treated initially with radiotherapy alone or radiotherapy and chemotherapy is insignificantly different, as stated above. And thirdly, it has been stated that the incidence of post treatment acute leukemia is higher in patients treated with a combined modality approach (4) than in patients treated with radiotherapy alone. For all these reasons, some workers have not considered initial combined modality treatment to be in the best interest of the patient.

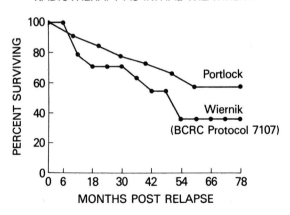

Figure 1

Alternative interpretation of the data may be appropriate. Figure 1 demonstrates that in both Portlock's study (3) and our own (2), there is a steady increase in the number of deaths in patients who have been treated with post-relapse "salvage" combination chemotherapy. The best interpretation of the data is that 40-60% of such patients will be permanently salvaged. Another interpretation is that the plateau at the end of the curve represents a computational rather than a biologic phenomenon and that it will become less prominent with the passage of time, as more patients are followed longer.

The concern about the development of post treatment acute leukemia in Hodgkin's disease patients is legitimate. However, a close analysis of the data (5-7) will reveal that while intensive combined modality treatment may be associated with a higher incidence of secondary acute leukemia than either modality alone, the incidence is highest in patients who receive the intensive modalities separated by considerable time (months or years) and receive both modalities when suffering from active Hodgkin's disease. Thus, the treatment situation most likely to result in secondary acute leukemia is initial intensive extended field radiotherapy followed by combination chemotherapy for relapse in the future, i.e. salvage therapy.

It should be emphasized at this point that even when one takes into consideration deaths from acute leukemia and other causes, and the success of combination chemotherapy for radiotherapy failure, the overall results are better in both the Stanford and Baltimore NCI study for patients initially treated with combined modality therapy compared to radiation therapy alone (1,2). As might have been suspected all along, it is probably better to remain free of Hodgkin's disease than to relapse with it.

How then does one explain the fact that in the Stanford study there is little overall survival difference between the combined modality and radiotherapy alone groups? Many of the patients in that study had prednisone omitted from the adjuvant chemotherapy which may have rendered that therapy less effective than MOPP (8). Two combined modality patients of 116 in the last Stanford report were found to have diffuse histiocytic lymphoma at autopsy and an additional 10 patients who died had no evidence of Hodgkin's disease at death (1). The inclusion of these 12 patients in the analysis of the data allows for the most conservative interpretation of the data but may not allow for a proper answer to the question of how to treat Hodgkin's disease. Furthermore, the Stanford reports are composite reports encompassing several similar studies. New patients have been entered over long periods of time. The constant infusion of new patients into the survival curves resulting from these studies tends to minimize the differences in the tails of the curves. This difficulty might be overcome by applying log-rank analysis to the data (9).

Finally, differences between the Stanford data and our own might be accounted for by different proportions of subgroups of patients in the two studies. We reported that patients with limited extranodal extension of Hodgkin's disease into lung tissue (Stages IIA_E, IIB_E, $IIIA_E$) have a very poor prognosis after radiotherapy alone but not after combined modality treatment (10,11). The high relapse rate of such patients was confirmed by Torti, et al (12) but they again found no survival advantage for the combined modality group. Others (13), however, have reported that patients with large mediastinal masses do more poorly than similarly staged patients without large mediastinal masses when treatment consists of radiotherapy alone, and others (14,15) have indicated that combined modality treatment is more successful in such patients. Since most patients with E stage of the lung have large mediastinal masses (11), it is likely that we and others (13-15) have identified a similar group of patients with a high likelihood of relapse and eventual death from Hodgkin's disease after initial treatment with radiotherapy alone.

We (16) and others (17,18) have also identified a subset of patients with Stage IIIA disease with a poor prognosis when initial treatment consists of radiotherapy alone. Such patients have lower intra-abdominal nodal disease rather than disease confined within the abdomen to the spleen and/or upper abdominal nodes. The latter patients (designated III_1A) have a prognosis similar to IIA patients without large mediatinal masses or E stage of the lung. Patients with lower abdominal nodal involvement (designated III_2A) were reported by us to fare better with combined modality treatment (16) and a recent cooperative study performed by our group, Vanderbilt University School of Medicine, the University of Chicago Cancer Research Center and the Harvard Medical School has confirmed the superior disease free and total survival for Stage III_2A patients treated initially with combined modality treatment (19).

On the basis of the above considerations, the Hodgkin's disease staging system detailed in Table 1 is proposed. This system groups patients according to what is likely to be optimal therapy.

Table 1

PROPOSED CLASSIFICATION AND TREATMENT RECOMMENDATIONS
OF HODGKIN'S DISEASE

Proposed New Stage	Ann Arbor Stage	Recommended Treatment
I	IA, IIA, III_1A (spleen and/or upper abdominal nodes represent only intra-abdominal involvement). Patients must have no mediastinal mass, or a mediastinal mass >1/3 the diameter of the chest. No E stage of lung (may be E stage elsewhere, such as thyroid, bone, etc).	Extended field radiotherapy alone - Pelvic nodes need not be treated.[34]
II	Any I, II, or IIIA patient with E stage of lung or mediastinal mass >1/3 chest diameter. All IB and IIB. All III_2A (lower abdominal node involvement).	Extended field radiotherapy followed by 6 courses of MOPP. Pelvic nodes irradiated only for III_2A.
III	IIIB, IVA, IVB	MOPP alone

COMPLICATIONS OF TREATMENT

Several decades of radiotherapy as the standard treatment for Hodgkin's disease have allowed the long term observation of many disease free patients for long term complications of treatment. The major complications that have been observed fall into several categories: endocrine, cardiovascular, pulmonary, and reproductive.

Endocrine complications

The most significant endocrine complication of radiotherapy for Hodgkin's disease is hypothyroidism (20). This complication may not develop for many years after the completion of treatment and usually presents in a subtle fashion. Chemical evidence of hypothyroidism is found in many patients in the absence of clinical evidence of the problem. Often chemical evidence of a hypofunctioning thyroid gland is accompanied by elevated blood TSH levels, a situation known to facilitate the development of thyroid carcinoma (21). It has been recommended, therefore, that replacement thyroid hormone be administered to such patients prophylactically even if no clinical signs of hypothyroidism are present.

Cardiovascular complications

A small but definite fraction of Hodgkin's disease patients who receive irradiation to the entire cardiac silhouette develop radiation-related pericarditis. The pericarditis usually spontaneously resolves, but it may occasionally become chronic and constrictive, and require pericardiectomy (22). In addition, reports of relatively young patients with Hodgkin's disease treated with radiotherapy subsequently dying of myocardial infarction have begun to appear (23). At autopsy, coronary artery intimal proliferation consistent with radiation damage has been determined to be the cause of the coronary occlusion in some cases (23).

Pulmonary complications

Most patients who have received mediastinal irradiation for large mediastinal masses have some permanent evidence of minimal to moderate pulmonary fibrosis on subsequent chest radiographs (24). While few patients have clinically evident pulmonary dysfunction associated with irradiation, prospective long term studies of pulmonary function in such patients have only recently been reported. do Pico et al (25) reported that in the year following upper mantle radiation therapy, significant declines in diffusing capacity for carbon monoxide, vital capacity, and inspiratory capacity usually occur. While these changes were transient and subclinical in most cases, in some they were prolonged, severe, and rarely fatal.

Reproductive dysfunction

Many patients who undergo pelvic irradiation for Hodgkin's disease, especially women, are rendered sterile by the treatment. While oophoropexy performed at staging laparotomy has reduced the incidence of female sterility (26), a significant incidence of sterility and menstrual dysfunction which tends to remain permanent is still observed.

Combination chemotherapy sequelae

The toxic effects of combination chemotherapy tend to be acute and to resolve with time. While many patients of both sexes are temporarily rendered sterile by MOPP chemotherapy, recent evidence documents that many such patients regain fertility months to years after the cessation of therapy (2,27). The incidence of second malignancies in patients so treated appears to be no greater than those observed with radiotherapy alone (28).

THOUGHTS FOR THE FUTURE

MOPP combination chemotherapy has been eminently successful in advanced Hodgkin's disease (29), especially in patients without symptoms (30). The above toxicity considerations coupled with the fact that radiotherapy alone is relatively poor treatment for certain subgroups of patients with early stage Hodgkin's disease dictate that alternate treatments for early stage disease be explored. The augmentation of results achieved in early stage disease by combined modality therapy provides evidence for the activity of MOPP combination chemotherapy in Hodgkin's disease confined primarily to lymph nodes. It is, therefore, appropriate to ask whether the superior results achieved with combined modality treatment compared to radiotherapy alone might be achieved with MOPP chemotherapy alone. Some pilot data attest to the efficacy of MOPP chemotherapy alone in early stage Hodgkin's disease. Ziegler and associates were able to achieve results comparable to radiotherapy in African children with early stage Hodgkin's disease using MOPP alone (31). In addition, the NCI experience with Stage IIIA disease treated with MOPP alone (30) is identical to that of others using combined modality therapy. We have recently demonstrated in a prospective, randomized trial that the complete response rate in patients with early stage disease is identical with combined modality therapy or MOPP alone (32). It is too early to evaluate remission duration differences, if any, in that study, however.

While MOPP chemotherapy may conceivably be proven to be optimal therapy for some patients with early stage Hodgkin's disease there are reasons to believe that combined modality treatment may ultimately prove to be optimal treatment for many. There is some evidence that nodular sclerosing Hodgkin's disease responds less well to chemotherapy than other histologic types (30). There is also evidence that patients wtih symptoms ascribable to Hodgkin's disease are less well treated with chemotherapy than asymptomatic patients (30). Therefore, early stage patients with symptoms ("B" disease) may fare better with combined modality treatment. There is some evidence that this is true for Stage IIIB patients (Ann Arbor Classification) (33). Finally, most tumors that are responsive to chemotherapy demonstrate an inverse relationship between bulk and response completeness and duration. This observation suggests that patients with large mediastinal masses may not do well with drugs alone.

The investigation of the treatment problems discussed above may ultimately lead to more precise and effective treatment for Hodgkin's disease by maximizing response rates and minimizing long term complications.

REFERENCES

1. Rosenberg, SA, HS Kaplan, E Glatstein, and CS Portlock, The role of adjuvant MOPP in the radiation therapy of Hodgkin's disease: A progress report after eight years on the Stanford trials. In: Adjuvant Therapy of Cancer, Salmon SS, and SE Jones (eds), North Holland, p 505-516, 1977

2. Wiernik, PH, J Gustafson, SC Schimpff, and C Diggs, Combined modality treatment of Hodgkin's disease confined to lymph nodes: results eight years later. Am J Med (in press) 1979

3. Portlock, CS, SA Rosenberg, E Glatstein, and MS Kaplan, Impact of salvage treatment on initial relapses in patients with Hodgkin's disease, Stages I-III. Blood 51: 825-833, 1978

4. Coleman, CN, CJ Williams, A Flint, et al, Hematologic neoplasia in patients treated for Hodgkin's disease. New Engl J Med 297: 1249-1252, 1977

5. Cadman, EC, RL Capizzi and JR Bertino, Acute nonlymphocytic leukemia. A delayed complication of Hodgkin's disease therapy: Analysis of 109 cases. Cancer 40: 1280-1296, 1977

6. Cavallin-Stähl, E, T Landberg, Z Ottow, and F Mitelman, Hodgkin's disease and acute leukaemia. Scand J Hematol 19: 273-280, 1977

7. Dick, FR, RD Maca, and R Hankenson, Hodgkin's disease terminating in a T-cell immunoblastic leukemia. Cancer 42: 1325-1329, 1978

8. British National Lymphoma Investigation: Value of prednisone in combination chemotherapy of Stage IV Hodgkin's disease. Br Med J 3: 413-414, 1975

9. Peto, R, MC Pike, P Armitage, NE Breslow, et al, Design and analysis of randomized clinical trials requiring prolonged observation of each patient. II Analysis and Examples. Brit J Cancer 35: 1-39, 1977

10. Levi, JA and PH Wiernik, Limited extranodal Hodgkin's disease: Unfavorable prognosis and therapeutic implications. Am J Med 63: 365-372, 1977

11. Levi, JA, PH Wiernik, and MJ O'Connell, Patterns of relapse in stages I, II and IIIA Hodgkin's disease: Influence of initial therapy and implications for the future. Int J Rad Oncol 2: 853-862, 1977

12. Torti, FM, CS Portlock, SA Rosenberg, and HS Kaplan, Extranodal (E) lesions in Hodgkin's disease (HD): Prognosis and response to therapy. Proc Amer Soc Clin Oncol 19: 367, 1978

13. Mauch, P, R Goodman, and S Hellman, The significance of mediastinal involvement in early stage Hodgkin's disease. Cancer 42: 1039-1045, 1978

14. Lange, B, P Littman, L Schnaufer, and A Evans, Treatment of advanced Hodgkin's disease in pediatric patients. Cancer 42: 1141-1145, 1978

15. Timothy, AR, SBJ Sutcliffe, AG Stanafeld, et al, Radiotherapy in the treatment of Hodgkin's disease. Br Med J 1: 1216-1249, 1978

16. Levi, JA, and PH Wiernik, The therapeutic implications of splenic involvement in Stage IIIA Hodgkin's disease. Cancer 39: 2158-2165, 1977

17. Desser, RK, HM Golomb, JE Ultmann, et al, Prognostic classification of Hodgkin's disease in pathologic stage III, based on anatomic considera- tion. Blood 49: 883-893, 1977

18. Stein, R, RM Hilborn, JM Flexner, et al, Anatomical substages of stage III Hodgkin's disease. Cancer 42: 429-436, 1978

19. Stein, RS, HM Golomb, CH Diggs, et al, Anatomical substages of stage III Hodgkin's disease: A collaborative study. N Engl J Med (in press) 1979

20. Schimpff, SC, PH Wiernik, J Wiswell, and P Salvatore, Radiation-related thyroid dysfunction: Implications for the treatment of Hodgkin's disease. Ann Intern Med (in press)

21. Doniach, I, The effect of radioactive iodine alone and in combination with methylthiouracil and acetylaminofluorene upon tumor production in the rat's thyroid gland. Br J Cancer 4: 223-234, 1950

22. Martin, RG, JC Ruckdeschel, P Chang, et al, Radiation-related peri- carditis. Amer J Cardiol 35: 216-220, 1975

23. McReynolds, RA, GL Gold, and WC Roberts, Coronary heart disease after mediastinal irradiation for Hodgkin's disease. Amer J Med 60: 39-45, 1976

24. Libshitz, HI, AB Brosof, and ME Southard, Radiographic appearance of the chest following extended field radiation therapy for Hodgkin's disease. Cancer 32: 206-215, 1973

25. doPico GA, AL Wiley Jr, P Rao, and MA Dicksie, Pulmonary reaction to upper mantle radiation therapy for Hodgkin's disease. Chest 75:688- 692, 1979

26. Ray, GR, HW Trueblood, and LP Enright, Oophoropexy: a means of preserving ovarian function following pelvic megavoltage radiotherapy for Hodgkin's disease. Radiol 96: 175-180, 1970

27. Sherins, RJ, and VT DeVita Jr, Effect of drug treatment for lymphoma on male reproductive capacity. Ann Int Med 79: 216-220, 1973

28. Arseneau, JC, RW Sponzo, DL Levin, et al, Nonlymphomatous malignant tumors complicating Hodgkin's disease. Possible association with intensive therapy. N Engl J Med 287: 1119-1122, 1972

29. DeVita, VT, AA Serpick, and PP Carbone, Combination chemotherapy in the treatment of advanced Hodgkin's disease. Ann Intern Med 73: 881-895, 1970

30. DeVita, V, GP Cannellos, S Hubbard, et al, Chemotherapy of Hodgkin's disease (HD) with MOPP: A 10 year progress report. Proc Amer Soc Clin Oncol 17: 269, 1976

31. Owen, CML, E Katongole-Mbidde, C Küre, et al, Childhood Hodgkin's disease in Uganda: A ten year experience. Cancer 42: 787-792, 1978

32. Wiernik, PH, RG Slawson, LC Burks, and CH Diggs: A randomized trial of radiotherapy (RT) and MOPP (c) vs. MOPP alone for stages IB-IIIA Hodgkin's disease. Proc Amer Soc Clin Oncol 20: (in press) 1979

33. Hoppe, RT, CS Portlock, E Glatstein, et al, Alternating chemotherapy and irradiation in the treatment of advanced Hodgkin's disease. Cancer 43: 472-481, 1979

34. Goodman, RL, AJ Piro, and S Hellman, Can pelvic irradiation be omitted in patients with pathologic stages IA and IIA Hodgkin's disease? Cancer 37: 2834-2839, 1976

THE ROLE OF RADIATION THERAPY IN THE MANAGEMENT OF CANCER OF THE HEAD AND NECK

Ralph M. Scott

Department of Radiation Therapy

University of Maryland Hospital

Baltimore, Maryland

INTRODUCTION

The role of radiotherapy in the management of cancer of the head and neck has undergone significant changes in the past decade promising to bring better recovery and survival. Largely, these changes have resulted from a better understanding of the response of normal tissue and tumors to ionizing irradiation and the increased awareness of the value of a multidisciplinary approach to the management of patients suffering from these diseases. Surgery and radiotherapy remain as the potentially curative methods available in the management of head and neck cancer, but chemotherapy is assuming an increasingly important role. In most sites stage I and stage II disease will yield to surgical excision or irradiation in an equally high percentage of cases, the treatment advantage going to the method resulting in the best cosmetic and functional result.

THERAPEUTIC ALTERNATIVES ACCORDING TO SITE

Oral Cavity

Small primary tumors in the oral cavity can be irradiated or resected successfully with little cosmetic or functional loss. More extensive disease usually is best managed by combined treatment consisting of surgery and preoperative or postoperative irradiation. This is especially true where bone involvement is present, since this predisposes to failure and an increased number of complications. Radical neck dissection or neck irradiation is always a consideration, and these methods may be complementary. When radical neck dissection is done and there are positive nodes in the histological specimen, recurrence rates exceed 50%, but this drops to less than 10% with preoperative or postoperative irradiation pointing out the value of combined modality treatment.

Paranasal Sinuses

Even in the early stages, cancer of the paranasal sinus is seldom seen without bone involvement, and combined modality treatment is usually most effective in patients with this disease. Small residual foci of cancer in bone is a common postoperative finding. When irradiating this site, inclusion of the ipsilateral eye in the beam is often necessary after irradiation. Orbital exenteration may be advisable since the sight usually will be lost due to cataract formation, and the eye will be subject to other problems including corneal ulceration, cataracts, and retinal damage.

Nasopharynx

In nasopharyngeal cancers, anatomic considerations dictate treatment by irradiation including the primary site and nodes. Because of the proximity to the base of the skull and its frequent involvement by tumor, plus the inaccessibility of the retropharyngeal nodes, surgical excision is not feasible and irradiation is needed for local control.

Oropharynx

Anatomic factors at this site also dispose for irradiation of early oropharyngeal cancer cases. Cure rates for irradiation are comparable to those obtained by surgery, and the functional impairment is usually less with the former treatment. Combined irradiation and surgery is better for the late stage cases where either modality alone is likely to fail. Nodal metastases are common from these sites and must always be considered in the treatment plan.

Hypopharynx

In hypopharyngeal cancer, pharyngolaryngectomy or irradiation alone have high local failure rates. Surgical removal, combined with preoperative or post-operative irradiation, gives the best results. Nodal metastases are very common in these patients and, even if not clinically evident, elective treatment of the neck is indicated to treat the microdeposits of tumor.

Glottis

In both glottic and supraglottic cancer, irradiation, by virtue of its lesser morbidity, is best in early stage disease. In subglottic tumors or glottic tumors with subglottic extension, combined surgery and irradiation is more likely to succeed. Advanced glottic and supraglottic tumors call for a total laryngectomy combined with irradiation which should include the neck nodes.

Salivary Glands

The treatment of salivary gland tumors is primarily surgical. Radiotherapy is indicated for residual or recurrent disease where it may improve salvage rates or attempt to control inoperable disease.

Other General Approaches

Chemotherapy may be of value in any of these tumor sites and has been particularly applied in late stage disease. Recently it has been applied earlier where it may be useful in controlling the primary disease prior to irradiation or against potential or actual distant spread. Immuno-stimulation is being explored, and it too may assume a significant role.

EQUIPMENT FOR RADIOTHERAPY

The multiplicity of anatomic sites of origin and pathological conditions encountered in the head and neck region call for a full range of radiotherapy equipment, including orthovoltage, often with peroral cones, interstitial implants using radium or other radionuclides, megavoltage or gamma ray external beam therapy, and electron beam therapy. Newer methods of irradiation with neutron beams, negative pi mesons and other particulate irradiation with their potential radiobiological and/or physical advantages may prove to have a place. With the aid of simulators and computers, treatment planning and dosimetry have become more precise, and CAT scanners may add to this precision.

FACTORS DETERMINING RESPONSE TO RADIOTHERAPY

Anoxia

In the 1950's, some very significant findings influenced our concepts of radiosensitivity. First, Read (1, 2) found that radiation sensitivity depended upon the presence of molecular oxygen in the tissues. Tomlinson and Gray (3) then established that there are foci of necrosis in tumors resulting from anoxia. Following this came the work of Puck and Marcus (4) on survival curves of irradiated mammalian cells showing an exponential relationship between survival and dose. Present concepts of radiosensitivity largely have evolved from these discoveries.

Approaches to deal with the anoxia problem have included the use of irradiation under hyperbaric oxygenation, the use of high linear energy transfer (LET), particle irradiation, the use of anoxic sensitizers, and hyperthermia. The irradiation of patients in hyperbaric oxygen has had a fair trial and has not proved to be of significant value. Clinical trials with neutron beam irradiation, which has a low oxygen enhancement ratio, have been underway for some time. In addition to the reduced oxygen-dependence with these and other high LET particles, there is also a decreased variation in response through the cell cycle and a lessened capacity for repair of cellular damage. Catteral (5) reports increasing rates of control using this method. Investigators in this country have met with less success; but so far, all their neutron beam therapy has been done on physics-oriented cyclotrons under less than optimal clinical conditions. Hospital based, medically dedicated units are planned and merit a trial. Negative pi mesons and heavy ions have possible dosimetric and radiobiological advantages, but are tremendously expensive to produce and, as yet, are not ready for routine clinical use.

The use of anoxic sensitizers is being explored. These compounds share with oxygen the property of setting the stage for free radical production, and thus hold the promise of minimizing the oxygen effect and the reason for failure in the irradiation of hypoxic tumors. They appear promising, but less toxic derivatives are needed if these agents are to be of significant value.

Hyperthermia as an adjunct to ionizing radiation has considerable promise and is being investigated. When used alone, it exerts a tumorcidal effect and appears to have a synergistic effect with irradiation and chemotherapy.

Size and Origin of Tumors

The tissue of origin and tumor size are important factors. In general, the sensitivity of tumors follows the sensitivity of the tissue from which they originate. For example, epithelial tumors, including squamous cell carcinomas and various adenocarcinomas which originate in the glandular tissue in the head and neck region, are about equal in their responsiveness to irradiation. The lymphomas are somewhat more sensitive. Size is very significant. Microscopic foci of disease respond to relatively small doses of radiation, but as tumor size increases so does the radiation dose required for control. Anoxic components of the tumors are size-related, in part, making the tumor less responsive to irradiation. Response of both tumors and normal tissue follows a sigmoid curve. As applied to human cancer, irradiation is most effective in small tumors. As tumor volume increases, so does the necessary dose until normal tissue tolerance is exceeded and complication rates become unacceptable. In some patients, this may be minimized or avoided in various ways such as decreasing the portal size as tumor size decreases and the use of interstitial radionuclides and/or small external field boosting doses to residual foci of disease. This is a common practice today.

LOCAL FAILURE OF TREATMENT

Surgical failure of head and neck cancer is usually the result of tumor left at the resected margins, sub-clinical spread or lymph node metastasis beyond the surgical field and local or bloodstream seeding by blood vessel invasion, or tumor manipulation at surgery. When stage III and stage IV lesions are surgically removed, there is a greater than 50% chance of recurrence above the clavical. Those with nodes not only have a high rate of local recurrence, but a 30-40% chance of distant metastasis, as well. Radiotherapy fails locally where the dose required exceeds tissue tolerance and, as with surgery, when there is disease present beyond the irradiated areas.

COMBINED MODALITY TREATMENT

General Considerations

Until recently, combined modality treatment was not commonly considered. When surgery or irradiation was chosen, the other modality was usually reserved for attempted salvage of cases having failed initial treatment. Less than radical surgery was not acceptable, and the all-or-none concept of radiation dose was widely held. Nodes were felt to be more resistant than the primary, and prophylactic neck irradiation was rarely done. The importance of anoxic foci in tumors as a function of their size, growth rate, tumor characteristics (exophytic or endophytic), and the tumor bed was not fully appreciated.

In the past, radiotherapists were attracted by chemotherapeutic agents, which might be synergistic or additive to irradiation, but their value in reducing tumor volume was not fully appreciated. Distant spread of head and neck cancer formerly was thought to be rare, and the need for systemic treatment was not recognized until recently when more late stage disease has been locally controlled, and distant disease become more evident.

Radiotherapy and Surgery

While surgery or irradiation will usually suffice in early stage disease; in late cases, the exclusive use of either, alone, often results in local or regional failure. Evidence has now been accumulated which strongly suggests that combined modality therapy can improve local control rates and function, and cosmesis as well. In the past, when preoperative or postoperative irradiation was used, it was combined with radical surgery. Now it appears that the integration of less radical surgical procedures with modest doses of irradiation may be better in some instances, both with regard to increasing survival and decreasing treatment sequelae and functional deficiencies. This does not mean that the surgical procedure should merely remove bulky areas of tumor. It should encompass all gross tumor at the primary site and remove all nodes which are grossly positive. The first echelon of lymph nodes for the primary lesion also should be removed, even though not grossly positive. The dose of irradiation then needed to control remaining cancer, as discussed, will be lower, reducing the incidence of serious sequelae.

Indications for combined treatment for primary tumors include those patients where cure rates by either mode alone are low, in high-grade tumors or tumors with a high tendency to vascular invasion, patients with known residual disease after either method of treatment alone, and patients having the possibility of decreased morbidity by less radical application of surgery and irradiation.

Indications for combined treatment of nodal metastasis include patients with multiple nodes, those with nodes larger than 2 cm., those with a high risk sub-clinical disease, and patients with nodes inaccessible to surgical removal.

Radiation and Chemotherapy

Chemotherapy now may be used before radiation to produce maximal tumor regression aiding in local control, during irradiation for synergistic or added effect, and after irradiation for the control of sub-clinical or clinical disease, both local and distant. With stage III and stage IV disease having an instance of distant metastasis approaching 40%, this is a worthwhile goal. Surgery and radiotherapy are only local methods of treatment and integration of chemotherapy with these has the potential, not only of local benefit, but for controlling early foci of metastatic disease, as well. Bleomycin, methotrexate, and cis-platinum have given encouraging preliminary results in this regard and are discussed by Muggia and Rosenzweig elsewhere in this publication. Randomized clinical trials are underway to evaluate the integration of these three modalities.

SUMMARY

With surgery, irradiation, and chemotherapy all having a vital role in the management of patients with cancer of the head and neck, the necessity for a team approach is apparent. Not only surgical, medical and radiation oncologists are involved; the team must also include social workers, speech therapists, maxilofacial prosthodontists, nutritionists, and others. The benefit derived from such cooperative practice is a major advance in head and neck cancer and will lead to improved survival, as well as improved cosmesis and function.

REFERENCES

1. Read, J, Mode of action of x-ray doses given with different oxygen concentrations. Brit J Radiol 25:336, 1952

2. Read, J, The effect of ionizing radiations on the broad beam root X. The dependence of the x-ray sensitivity on disolved oxygen. Brit J Radiol 25:89-99, 1952

3. Tomlinson, RH and LH Gray, The histological structure of some human lung cancers and the possible implications for radiotherapy. Brit J Cancer 9:539, 1955

4. Puck, TT and PI Marcus, Action of x-rays on mammalian cells. J Exper Med 103:653-668, 1956

5. Catteral, M, DK Buley, and I Southerland, Second report on results of a randomized clinical trial of fast neutrons compared with X or gamma rays in the treatment of advanced tumors of the head and neck. Brit Med J 1:1642, 1977

6. Hussey, DH, RG Parker, and CC Rogers, A preliminary report of the fast neutron therapy pilot studies in the United States. In: Particle Radiation Therapy Proceedings of International Workshop. American College of Radiology 2:435-450, 1976

SYSTEMIC CHEMOTHERAPY IN
ADVANCED HEAD AND NECK CANCER

Franco M. Muggia and Marcel Rozencweig
National Cancer Institute
National Institutes of Health
Bethesda, Maryland

INTRODUCTION

The management of head and neck cancer will become an increasingly important problem for medical oncologists. Currently, chemotherapy is generally employed for tumors that are beyond the reach of surgery and radiotherapy. However, although a number of active compounds are available for use, the rapidly declining performance status of the patients and the lack of clearly evaluable lesions at this advanced stage of disease often hamper the rational administration of cytotoxic agents. For these reasons, chemotherapy is likely to become a common procedure during the initial phases of treatment over the next few years. As will be pointed out later, trials are already underway to define the role of chemotherapy under these favorable circumstances, termed the "initial curative approach".

In this review, we will first discuss published data on single and combination systemic chemotherapy regimens in the treatment of advanced disease, and then elaborate on specific areas worthy of further investigation.

SINGLE AGENT CHEMOTHERAPY

The systemic administration of single agents has elicited a wide range of response rates due, in large part, to variability in patient selection, response criteria, and methods of data reporting. The most consistent antitumor activity has been identified for three drugs: methotrexate, bleomycin, and, more recently, cis-diamminedichloroplatinum (II) (cis-platine). However, the relative usefulness and specificity for a particular site of origin or histologic type of squamous cell cancer has not been established for these drugs. With these limitations in mind, it is worth reviewing in detail the antitumor activity of these three agents, which form the basis for most chemotherapeutic approaches in these diseases.

Methotrexate

Methotrexate (MTX) is often referred to as the standard chemotherapeutic agent for the treatment of advanced squamous cell carcinoma of head and neck origin.

Since the initial recognition during the 1960's of its activity against these tumors, the drug has been widely explored with several modes of administration. Encouraging response rates have been commonly reported in large series using single intermittent IV treatments (table 1). Thus with weekly doses of 60 mg/m^2, Leone et al (3) obtained an overall response rate of 63% with complete tumor regressions noted in more than one half of the responders. Of note, the median response duration achieved in this study was similar for complete and partial remissions (17 versus 20 weeks).

Table 1. Single agent activity of systemic methotrexate

Investigator	Dose (mg/m^2)	Schedule	Route	No of Pts.	Response rate (%) Overall	Complete
Papac (1)	15*	Daily x 5 q 4 wks	PO	24	17	-
	25*	Daily x 5 q 4 wks	IV	23	17	-
Lane (2)	20-50*	q 4-7 days	IV	27	52	15
Leone (3)	60	Weekly	IV	30	63	33
Levitt (4)	80-200	30 hr q 2 wks	IV	16	44	-
	360-1080**	36-42 hr q 2 wks	IV	25	60	-

*Total dose per treatment
**Leucovorin rescue

More recently, interest in administering high doses of MTX, followed by citrovorum factor (CF) "rescue", has led to a proliferation of trials including MTX-CF in a variety of dose schedules. The rationale for clinically investigating these regimens is derived from experimental findings in the L1210 murine leukemia suggesting that the therapeutic index of MTX may be improved with MTX-CF at specified dose sequences (5). Higher doses of MTX could produce higher intracellular concentrations of free drug resulting in lethality to a larger number of malignant cells whereas toxic manifestations in normal target tissues would be safely reversed by selective CF rescue. Furthermore, the use of these high dose treatments could increase the likelihood that the drug actually reaches poorly vascular tumor areas. A number of these high-dose regimens with CF rescue have, in fact, achieved antitumor activity in head and neck cancer (6). Unfortunately, this treatment requires considerable experience and expense, and has not convincingly shown results superior to conventional dose schedules.

In a randomized study conducted by Levitt et al (4), patients received MTX alone given at maximally tolerated doses as 30-hr IV infusions or at higher doses followed by CF rescue and 36- to 42-hr IV infusions. These patients were unsuitable for radiation therapy or surgery, but none had received prior chemotherapy. The respective overall response rates were 44% for a median of 12 weeks versus 60% for a median of 11 weeks. Pronounced leukopenia was less frequently encountered with the high-dose regimen suggesting an improvement in the therapeutic index of methotrexate with CF rescue. In a large scale trial carried out by the Eastern Cooperative Oncology Group (7), 243 patients were randomly allocated to receive weekly MTX (40 mg/m^2) or biweekly MTX (240 mg/m^2) followed by CF rescue or a 3-drug combination including MTX. The study protocol called for dose escalation until toxicity or response occurred. This requirement was actually fulfilled in only 70% of the patients. A preliminary analysis of the data indicated an overall response rate of 24% among the 191 evaluated patients with no significant differences in response rate between the three treatment arms. However, firm conclusion on this trial must await the publication of the final report.

At this point, the optimum treatment with systemic high-dose MTX has not been clarified. There is no agreement on the magnitude of the dose or the duration of the infusion. The most appropriate rescue procedure is another problem that lacks a definite answer. In any event, the high-dose MTX approach remains an interesting experimental therapeutic concept, both in terms of increasing the therapeutic index and overcoming drug resistances to low dose. In this last respect, MTX is somewhat unique in the ability to safely deliver doses several logs higher, as long as one manipulates with extreme caution variables such as time of drug administration until CF rescue, absolute amount given and intensity of CF rescue.

Bleomycin

The role of bleomycin (BLM) in the treatment of head and neck cancer has been recently reviewed (8). As a single agent, the drug appears generally less effective than MTX but probable differences in trial design preclude meaningful comparisons in nonrandomized studies. The broad range of response rates reported with bleomycin illustrates the difficulties of accurately assessing the antitumor activity of cytotoxic agents especially in head and neck cancer. In large series, bleomycin has elicited response rates varying between 6 and 45% (table 2). Even with the highest overall figure, complete tumor regressions have been rarely encountered (9). Most of these data have been obtained in broad

Table 2. Single agent activity of systemic bleomycin

Investigator	Dose (mg/m^2)	Schedule	Route	No. of patients	Response rate (%) Overall	Complete
Halnan (9)	20*	Twice weekly	IV or IM	53	45	6
Bonadonna (10)	10, 15, 30 15, 30	Twice weekly Daily x 5-8	IV	48	38	4
Haas (11)	10	Twice weekly	IV vs IM	64	19	0
EORTC (12)	10-20 20	Daily x 10-38 Twice weekly	IV or IM	54	17	2
Yagoda (13)	9.25	Daily to toxicity	IV	46	13	-
Durkin (14)	10	Twice weekly	IV vs IM	81	6	1

*Total dose per treatment

phase II trials that included patients with undefined prognostic factors or with far advanced disease no longer suitable for standard therapy. Thus, bleomycin achieved a 6% overall response rate in a study reported by Durkin et al (14) but 25% of the patients in this study had pulmonary metastases, undoubtedly reflecting a very advanced stage of disease. In addition, this trial was restricted to previously treated patients refractory to all conventional treatment modalities, including chemotherapy.

The duration of responses to BLM has generally not exceeded 2-3 months. This short duration may have, in part, resulted from a selection of a poor risk population but also could be related to a limited treatment duration because of the cumulative toxicity of bleomycin.

An optimal mode of administering bleomycin remains to be determined. The route of administration, IV or IM, and the dose schedules investigated in large studies do not seem to strikingly influence response, but there is some suggestion that doses above 10 mg/m^2, daily or twice weekly, might be associated with higher response rates (table 2).

Experience with continuous infusions is presently limited despite a fair amount of available experimental information. In vitro studies of cell cycle specificity showed BLM to be most active on cells in mitosis or in G-2 phase (15). The reported cell cycle time for epidermoid tumors is between 25 and 48 hours (16). Bleomycin may be more effective on cells exposed to it for the duration of their cell cycle (17). Finally, there is experimental evidence that repeated drug administration at short intervals, and particularly continuous infusion therapy, may minimize repair mechanism after BLM-induced DNA damage (18).

Krakoff et al (19) reported the results of a broad phase I-II trial using continuous infusions of bleomycin at a daily dose of 0.02 to 0.50 mg/kg until limiting toxicity was apparent. Some of the patients in this trial had previously been treated with conventional IV push bleomycin. Eleven patients with head and neck cancer were adequately treated and two achieved partial remissions. Little information was provided concerning these patients or their treatment and, despite the relatively unfavorable results, additional studies of this mode of administration seem warranted in head and neck cancer.

Cis-diamminedichloroplatinum II

The antitumor properties of cis-diamminedichloroplatinum II (DDP) have been identified by Rosenberg et al (20). Preclinical studies showed that DDP was not schedule-dependent and exhibited synergism with irradiation and a variety of anticancer agents (21,22). As with MTX and BLM, its optimal administration is actively being explored particularly in patients afflicted with nutritional deficiencies and poor performance status. In fact, the potential of DDP was not appreciated until after investigators established that vigorous hydration permitted safe administration of doses that would ordinarily be nephrotoxic (23). Currently, additional manipulations of dose scheduling are taking place in an effort to circumvent the noticeable gastrointestinal intolerance of this agent.

DDP appears to have remarkable antitumor activity in head and neck cancer. The potential of DDP in the chemotherapy of this malignancy has been suggested by data obtained at Memorial Sloan-Kettering Cancer Center. First detected in an early clinical trial (24), the activity of the drug was subsequently documented in a pilot study using high doses of the drug with hyperhydration and mannitol diuresis (23). Twenty-six patients with far-advanced epidermoid head and neck cancer were treated with this high-dose regimen (25). All patients had previous radiotherapy and a majority of them also had surgery and/or chemotherapy. Two complete remissions for 2+ and 6+ months and 6 partial remissions for periods ranging from 1 to 8+ months were achieved. These investigators also explored a simplified weekly regimen (26). The drug was given at 40 mg/m^2 with no prehydration or forced diuresis. Tumor response was seen in 4 of 13 patients but dose-limiting nephrotoxicity developed in one half of the patients.

The therapeutic potential of DDP in the treatment of head and neck carcinoma has been confirmed in two other studies. The Southwest Oncology Group has developed an outpatient DDP program with monthly courses consisting of 50 mg/m^2 on days 1 and 8 (7). Twenty-six patients were analyzed in a preliminary report: 5 of these died within one month from tumor progression and 8 of the remaining patients achieved tumor regression. At Stanford, Jacobs et al used 24-hr infusions at a dose of 80 mg/m^2 with vigorous hydration but no mannitol (28). Of 18 patients, 7 experienced complete or partial remission. This mode of administration was reported to markedly circumvent the troublesome gastrointestinal toxicity of the drug.

Additional experience with DDP as single agent chemotherapy will probably be limited in head and neck cancer. In addition to its intrinsic antitumor effect, DDP does not produce mucositis and relatively little to moderate drug-induced myelosuppression is encountered. These features have prompted its rapid incorporation into combination chemotherapy regimens.

Other Drugs

Experience with other commercially available agents is quite scanty and has been essentially compiled from older series by Livingston and Carter (29). Promising activity was suggested with cyclophosphamide and hydroxyurea but these data were based on response criteria inappropriate by current standards. More solid data have been reported with vinblastine (30), but confirmation of these results is needed. The value of vincristine cannot yet be assessed in view of the limited information that is presently available (31). This compound has often been included in combinations based on its lack of hematologic toxicity, the reported toxicity of vinblastine, and tumor cell kinetic rationale (32). The performance of adriamycin has been generally disappointing when compared with its striking antitumor activity against many other malignancies (33-37). Nitrosoureas also appear poorly active (38).

Additional data are being accumulated with a number of investigational drugs (38). These results were primarily obtained in broad phase II studies which limits the conclusions that can be drawn regarding drug activity. Inhibitors of dihydrofolate reductase, such as DDMP and Baker's antifol, merit further attention in view of the activity of MTX, the preliminary activity of DDMP (39), and the potential for activity in MTX-resistant tumors.

COMBINATION CHEMOTHERAPY

At this time, there is little evidence that combination chemotherapy has been superior to single agents in yielding better or longer responses in advanced head and neck cancer. In addition, many combinations have been more toxic and less manageable than single agents in patients at these stages. However, it remains to be seen whether earlier use of drug treatment and exclusion of agents with borderline intrinsic activity will lead to more promising combination regimens. For the sake of brevity, only those regimens including BLM and MTX and the newer combinations including DDP have been reviewed.

Several 2-drug combinations employing BLM and MTX have been reported (table 3), but superiority of any of these treatments over each agent given alone has not been demonstrated. As one might expect, the dose-limiting toxicity is mucocutaneous. In addition, severe myelosuppression has been encountered, suggesting more than additive effects on the bone marrow. The incidence of pulmonary complications has also been higher than usually observed with bleomycin alone. Experience with sequential administration by Swiss investigators indicated severe myelosuppression when BLM was given at 30 mg twice weekly (42). At lower doses, on a weekly schedule, the combination was much

Table 3. Systemic combination chemotherapy with bleomycin (BLM) and methotrexate (MTX)

Investigator	IV DOSE		Schedule	No. of responses/ No. of evaluable patients*	Response duration (mos)
	BLM	MTX			
Medenica (40)	15 mg	0.6 mg/kg	Weekly	13/26 (0)	6
Bonadonna (41)	Unspecified	40 mg/m^2	Weekly	2/16 (-)	-
Broquet (42)	30 mg	0.4 mg/kg	Twice weekly	9/15 (0)	2-3.5
Yagoda (43)	15 units	15 mg/m^2	q 4-14 days	8/15 (3)	1-8+
Lokich (44)	10-15 mg/m^2	15-25 mg/m^2	Twice weekly	4/5 (1)	-
Mosher** (45)	105 mg	480 mg/m^2	Sequential	2/4 (-)	-

*( ) = No. of complete responders

**BLM given IM over 5 days every 12 days. MTX given over 36 hrs followed by citrovorum factor between BLM courses better tolerated, but the favorable response rate was maintained and the duration of response was longer (40).

Several combinations including MTX, BLM, and several additional agents, exclusive of DDP, have been investigated (table 4). Although the response rates appear generally higher than achieved with single agents, neither complete regressions nor response durations are particularly encouraging. Combinations, including only BLM and MTX, with other drugs, have not looked particularly impressive either.

Incorporation of DDP into several combinations has followed logically from its relative lack of myelosuppression and reproducible activity when used alone (table 5). However, combinations of DDP with MTX or with BLM must take into account possible compounding of toxicity by altering renal excretion of the latter two agents. Thus, great care must be taken in any attempts at combination chemotherapy that included drugs depending on renal excretion. The most extensive experience with DDP-containing combinations has been obtained by investigators at Memorial Sloan-Kettering Cancer Center. After a disappointing initial experience with lower doses of DDP and daily treatments with BLM (55), a study including 3 mg/kg of DDP followed by bleomycin (0.25 mg/kg/day) by continuous infusion on day 3 through 10 yielded 4 CR and 4 PR among 21 evaluable patients with no previously treated disease (56). More recently, Hong et al confirmed this experience in a similar setting and achieved 10 PR in 15 patients treated with an identical schedule (57). Recently, combinations including conventional dose MTX or HDMTX-CF and BLM-DDP have also been reported with interesting results. Difficulties in combining all three drugs have been encountered and some drug-related deaths have been reported with regimens including HDMTX-CF (63,64).

In conclusion, the exploration of new combinations including DDP appears warranted, but comparative trials against single agents will be required to definitely establish that we are not caught up in a wave of false enthusiasm.

Table 4. Systemic combination chemotherapy including bleomycin and methotrexate

Treatment	No. of Evaluable Patients	Response rate (%)		Duration (mos.)	Investigators
		Overall	Complete		
VCR-ADM-BLM-MTX-5FU-HYD-6MP	24	79	-	-	Price (46)
VCR-BLM-MTX	42	71	10	2.5-4	Pouillart (47) Ratkin (48)
BLM-MTX/BLM-HYD	17	59	-	1-8	Costanzi (49)
BLM-CTX-MTX-5FU	33	48	12	7	Stathopoulos (50), Cortes(51)
CTX-VCR-BLM/MTX/ADM MeCCNU	28	43	17	6	Livingston (52)
CTX-ADM-MTX-BLM	26	35	0	2.5	Wittes (53)
CTX-ADM-VCR-BLM/MTX-CTX-ADM	19	26	10	-	Murphy (54)

ADM = adriamycin; BLM = bleomycin; CTX = cytoxan; 5FU = 5-fluorouracil; HYD = hydroxyurea;
6 MP = 6-mercaptopurine; MTX = methotrexate; VCR = vincristine

Table 5. Systemic combination chemotherapy including DDP

Treatment	No. of Patients	No. of responses		Investigators
		All	Complete	
DDP-BLM	67	30	4	Wittes (55)
				Randolph (56)
				Hong (57)
				Bianco (58)
DDP-ADM	11	5	1	Bonomi (59)
DDP-VCR-BLM	16	6	0	Amer (60)
DDP-VCR-MTX	7	0		Bianco (58)
DDP-BLM-MTX	66	41	7	Kaplan (61)
				Caradonna (62)
				Elias (63)
				Wittes (64)
DDP-BLM-MTX-VLB	21	10	0	Wittes (64)

OTHER AREAS OF INVESTIGATION

Other areas relevant to the systemic therapy of head and neck cancer will be mentioned briefly, although each is worthy of separate analysis and discussion.

Immunotherapy

Immunotherapy has so far been disappointing in advanced disease patients. Various studies have included BCG and non-specific stimulation by MER-BCG. Interest has also developed in intralesional C. parvum.

Intraarterial (IA) Chemotherapy

IA chemotherapy has been extensively used in the past, particularly with MTX (65). However, little data are available to estimate the role of IA versus systemic chemotherapy in head and neck cancer since no comparative trial of the two modalities has been published. Overall, the IA procedure is associated with significant morbidity and a modest response rate, in spite of the relatively favorable prognosis of patients selected for this treatment modality. Studies with IA bleomycin have been published, but not with particularly striking results. An EORTC study comparing IA bleomycin and IA MTX is awaiting final analysis. Studies of other single agents, such as adriamycin and DTIC, given IA, are also in progress. Experience with drug combinations have also been reported but it is difficult to assess a distinct advantage over systemic administration.

Combined Radiotherapy and Chemotherapy

This approach has been extensively studied, but its impact has been difficult to assess (65). A controlled study, combining MTX and irradiation, by the Radiation Therapy Oncology Group (RTOG), suggested that chemotherapy might decrease the incidence of distant metastases (66). Favorable experience has also been reported in controlled studies with 5FU therapy confined to the oral cavity, and to the maxillary sinus, and in a small study with hydroxyurea in all sites. Negative experience with all these agents has also been reported. A difficulty in assessing these studies, of course, is the multitude of sites influencing prognosis of patients and the variety of local treatment techniques that are included. In addition, irradiation doses usually must be lowered because of additive toxicities to normal tissues. For these reasons, and perhaps because of the more reproducible activity of current chemotherapies, recent trends have favored a sequential trial design with chemotherapy preceding irradiaiton.

CONCLUSIONS

The role of chemotherapy is becoming better delineated in the treatment of head and neck cancer, and integration of this modality into initial treatment of the disease is now being achieved. Accordingly, the National Cancer Institute recently sponsored a protocol for evaluating the role of chemotherapy given prior to local interventions in patients with selected stages of the oral and laryngeal regions. This study with chemotherapy consisting of induction with BLM-DDP and maintenance DDP will soon be underway.

It is important to re-emphasize that there are many gaps in our knowledge of chemotherapy in this disease, i.e.,

1. The response rate according to disease site.
2. The relative efficacy of various agents.
3. The relative advantage of combination over single agent chemo-therapy.
4. The role of specialized techniques such as IA administration, chemo-immunotherapy, and scheduling of combinations and irradiation.

The achievements to date should serve as a stimulus for exploring the chemotherapeutic modality in a variety of clinical circumstances and stages. It is hoped that current approaches will lead to better local control and improvement in survival rates. Although not currently within reach, the prospect of diminishing the disfiguring and disabling impact of radical surgery must be the ultimate goal of systemic therapy.

REFERENCES

1. Papac, RJ, EM Jacobs, LV Foye Jr., et al, Systemic therapy with amethopterin in squamous carcinoma of the head and neck. Cancer Chemother Rep 32:47-54, 1963

2. Lane, M, JE Moore, III, H Levin, et al, Methotrexate therapy for squamous cell carcinomas of the head and neck. JAMA 204:561-564, 1968

3. Leone. LA, MM Albala, VB Rege, Treatment of carcinoma of the head and neck with intravenous methotrexate. Cancer 21:828-831, 1968

4. Levitt, M, MB Mosher, RC DeConti, et al, Improved therapeutic index of methotrexate with "leucovorin rescue". Cancer Res 33:1729-1734, 1973

5. Goldin, A, JM Venditti, SR Humphreys, et al, Studies on the management of mouse leukemia (L1210) with antagonists of folic acid. Cancer Res 15:742-747, 1955

6. Von Hoff, DD, M Rozencweig, AC Louie, et al, "Single"-agent activity of high-dose methotrexate with citrovorum factor rescue. Cancer Treat Rep 62:233-235, 1978

7. DeConti, RC, Phase III comparison of methotrexate with leucovorin vs methotrexate alone vs a combination of methotrexate plus leucovorin, cyclophosphamide and cytosine arabinoside in head and neck cancer. Prodeed Am Soc Clin Oncol 17:248, 1976

8. Turrisi, AT, III, M Rozencweig, DD Von Hoff, et al, the role of bleomycin in the treatment of advanced head and neck cancer. In: Bleomycin: Current Status and New Developments, Carter, SK, ST Crooke, H Umezawa (eds), New York, Academic Press, pp. 151-163, 1978

9. Halnan, KE, NM Bleehen, TB Brewin, et al, Early clinical experience with bleomycin in the United Kingdom in series of 105 patients. Brit Med J 4:635-638, 1972.

10. Bonadonna, G, M De Lena, S Monfardini, et al, Clinical trials with bleomycin in lymphomas and in solid tumors. Europ J Cancer 8:205-215, 1972

11. Haas, CD, CA Coltman Jr., JA Gottlieb, et al, Phase II evaluation of bleomycin. A Southwest Oncology Group study. Cancer 38:8-12, 1976

12. Clinical Screening Cooperative Group of the European Organization for Research on Treatment of Cancer: Study of the clinical efficiency of bleomycin in human cancer. Brit Med J 2:643-645, 1970

13. Yagoda, A, B Mukherji, C Young, et al, Bleomycin, an antitumor antibiotic. Clinical experience in 274 patients. Ann Intern Med 77:861-870, 1972

14. Durkin, WJ, AP Pugh, E Jacobs, et al, Bleomycin (NSC-125066) therapy of responsive solid tumors. Oncology 33:260-264, 1976

15. Barranco, SC, RM Humphrey, The effects of bleomycin on survival and cell progression in Chinese hamster cells in vitro. Cancer Res 31:1218-1223, 1971

16. Frindel, E, E Malaise, M Tubiana, Cell proliferation kinetics in five human solid tumors. Cancer 22:611-620, 1968

17. Drewinko, B, JK Novak, SC Barranco, The response of human lymphoma cells in vitro to bleomycin and 1, 3-bis (2-chloroethyl)-1-nitrosourea. Cancer Res 32:1206-1208, 1972

18. Takabe, Y, T Miyamoto, H Watanabe, et al, Bleomycin: mammalian cell lethality and cellular basis of optimal schedule. J Natl Cancer Inst 59:1251-1255, 1977

19. Krakoff, IH, E Cvitkovic, V Currie, et al, Clinical pharmacologic and therapeutic studies of bleomycin given by continuous infusion. Cancer 40:2927-2037, 1977

20. Rosenberg, B, L Van Camp, T. Krigas, Inhibition of cell division in Escherichia coli by electrolysis products from a platinum electrode. Nature (London) 205:698-699, 1965

21. Rozencweig, M, DD Von Hoff, M Slavik, et al, Cis-diamminedichloro-platinum (II): a new anticancer drug. Ann Intern Med 86:803-812, 1977

22. Muggia, FM, M Rozencweig, Platinum compounds in clinical oncology: review and future prospects. In: Advances in Cancer Chemotherapy, Carter, SK, A Goldin, K Kuretani, et al (eds), Baltimore, University Park Press, pp. 141-153, 1978

23. Hayes, DM, E Cvitkovic, RB Golbey, et al, High dose cis-platinum diammine dichloride. Cancer 39:1372-1381, 1977

24. Lippman, AJ, C Helson, J Helson, et al, Clinical trials of cis-diammine-dichloroplatinum (NSC-119875). Cancer Chemother Rep 57:191-200, 1973

25. Wittes, RE, E Cvitkovic, J Shah, et al, Cis-dichlorodiammineplatinum (II) in the treatment of epidermoid carcinoma of the head and neck. Cancer Treat Rep 61:359-366, 1977

26. Randolph, VL, RE Wittes, Weekly administration of cis-diamminedichloro-platinum (II) without hydration or osmotic diuresis. Europ J Cancer 14:753-756, 1978

84

27. Panettiere, FJ, M Lane, D Lehane, Effectiveness of a new outpatient program utilizing CACP in the chemotherapy of advanced epidermoid head and neck tumors. A SWOG study, Proceed Am Soc Clin Oncol 19:410, 1978

28. Jacobs, C, JR Bertino, DR Goffinet, et al, 24-hour infusion of cis-platinum in head and neck cancer. Cancer (in press)

29. Livingston, R, S Carter, Single Agents in Cancer Chemotherapy, New York, Plenum Press, 1970

30. Smart, CR, DB Rochlin, AM Nahum, et al, Clinical experience with vinblastine sulfate (NSC-49842) in squamous cell carcinoma and other malignancies. Cancer Chemother Rep 34:31-45, 1963

31. Livingston, RB, LH Einhorn, MA Burgess, et al, Advances in treatment of recurrent and disseminated squamous carcinoma of the lung, head and neck. In: Cancer Chemotherapy, Chicago, Yearbook Medical Publishers, pp. 233-249, 1975

32. Livingston, RB, GP Bodey, JA Gottlieb, et al, Kinetic scheduling of vincristine (NSC-67574) and bleomycin (NSC-125066) in patients with lung cancer and other malignant tumors. Cancer Chemother Rep 57:219-224, 1973

33. Dowell, KE, DM Armstrong, JB Aust, et al, Systemic chemotherapy of advanced head and neck malignancies. Cancer 35:1116-1120, 1975

34. Knight, EW, J Horton, C Reilly, et al, A comparison of weekly vs 3-week course adriamycin in solid tumors. Proceed Am Assoc Cancer Res 13:92, 1972

35. Benjamin, RS, PH Wiernik, NR Bachur, Adriamycin chemotherapy. Efficacy, safety, and pharmacologic basis of an intermittent single high-dosage schedule. Cancer 33:19-27, 1974

36. Bonadonna, G, G Beretta, G Tancini, et al, Adriamycin (NSC-123127) studies at the Istituto Nazionale Tumori, Milan. Cancer Chemother Rep 6:231-245, 1975

37. Krakoff, IH, Adriamycin (NSC-123127) studies in adult patients. Cancer Chemother Rep 6:253-257, 1975

38. Rozencweig, M, DD Von Hoff, FM Muggia, Investigational chemo-therapeutic agents in head and neck cancer. Sem Oncol 4:425-429, 1977

39. Alberto, P, R Peytremann, R Medenica, et al, Clinical experience with a combination of DDMP, a diaminopyrimidine, and folinic acid (CF). Proceed Am Soc Clin Oncol 19:346, 1978

40. Medenica, R, P Alberto, W Lehmann, Traitement des carcinomes epidermoides oro-pharyngo-larynges dissemines par combinaison de methotrexate et de bleomycine a petites doses. Schewiz Med Woschr 106:799-802, 1976

41. Bonadonna, G, G Tancini, E Bajetta, Controlled studies with bleomycin in solid tumors and lymphomas. Prog Biochem Pharmacol 11:172-184, 1976

42. Broquet, MA, E Jacot-Descombe, A Montandon, et al, Traitement des carcinomes epidermoides oto-pharyngo-larynges par combinaision de methotrexate et de bleomycine. Schweiz Med Woschr 104:18-22, 1974

43. Yagoda, A, AJ Lippman, RJ Winn, et al, Combination chemotherapy with bleomycin (BLM) and methotrexate (MTX) in patients with advanced epidermoid carcinomas. Proceed Am Soc Clin Oncol 16:247, 1975

44. Lokich, JJ, E Frei III, Phase II study of concurrent methotrexate and bleomycin chemotherapy. Cancer Res 34:2240-2242, 1974

45. Mosher, MB, RC DeConti, JR Bertino, Bleomycin therapy in advanced Hodgkin's disease and epidermoid cancers. Cancer 30:56-60, 1972

46. Price, LA, BT Hill, AH Calvert, et al, Kinetically-based multiple drug treatment for advanced head and neck cancer. Brit Med J 3:10-11, 1975

47. Pouillart, P, G Mathe, Bleomycin in rational combinations of chemotherapy. GANN monograph on cancer research No 19, Fundamental and clinical studies of bleomycin, Univ Tokyo Press, pp. 279-283, 1976

48. Ratkin, GA, CA Brown, JH Ogura, Combination chemotherapy in head and neck cancer. Proceed Am Soc Clin Oncol 19:330, 1978

49. Costanzi, JJ, D Loukas, RG Gagliano, et al, Intravenous bleomycin infusion as a potential synchronizing agent in human disseminated malignancies. A preliminary report. Cancer 38:1503-1506, 1976

50. Stathopoulas, G, E Wiltshaw, LA Price, Quadruple chemotherapy in advanced squamous cell carcinoma of the head and neck. Brit J Clin Pract 30:188-189, 1976

51. Cortes, EP, VC Amin, R Khafif, et al, Bleomycin (B) infusion with cyclophosphamide (C), methotrexate (M) and 5-fluorouracil (F) in previously irradiated head and neck cancer. Proceed Am Assoc Cancer Res 19:140, 1978

52. Livingston, RB, LH Einhorn, MA Burgess, et al, Sequential combination chemotherapy for advanced, recurrent squamous carcimona of the head and neck. Cancer Treat Rep 60:103-105, 1976

86

53. Wittes, RE, RH Spiro, J Shah, et al, Chemotherapy of head and neck cancer: combination treatment with cyclophosphamide, adriamycin, methotrexate and bleomycin. Med Ped Oncol 3:301-309, 1977

54. Murphy, WK, RB Livingston, E Gehan, et al, Sequential chemotherapy in the treatment of cancer of the head and neck. Proceed Am Assoc Cancer Res 18:190, 1977

55. Wittes, RE, F Brescia, CW Young, et al, Combination chemotherapy with cis-diamminedichloroplatinum (II) and bleomycin in tumors of the head and neck. Oncology 32:202-207, 1975

56. Randolph, VL A Vallejo, RH Spiro, et al, Combination therapy of advanced head and neck cancer: induction of remissions with diamminedichloroplatinum (II), bleomycin, and radiation therapy. Cancer 41:460-467, 1978

57. Hong, WK, R Bhutani, S Shapshay, et al, Induction chemotherapy of advanced unresectable head and neck cancer with cis-diammine dichloro platinum (II) (DDP) and bleomycin. Proceed Am Soc Clin Oncol 19:321, 1978

58. Bianco, AA, SG Taylor IV, SD Reich, et al, Combination chemotherapy in head and neck squamous cancer. Proceed Am Soc Clin Oncol 19:380, 1978

59. Bonomi, PD, J Mladineo, GD Wilbanks, et al, Phase II trial of adriamycin and cis-diamminedichloroplatinum (CACP) in advanced squamous cell carcinoma (SCC). Proceed Am soc Clin Oncol 18:311, 1977

60. Amer, MH, R Izbicki, M Al-Sarraf, Combination of high dose cis-platinum, oncovin and bleomycin (COB) in treatment of patients with advanced head and neck cancer. Proceed Am Soc Clin Oncol 19:312, 1978

61. Kaplan, BH, SE Vogl, Methotrexate (M), bleomycin (B) and diamminedichloroplatinum (D) in squamous cancers (Sq Ca) of the head and neck, cervix and other sites. Proceed Am Soc Clin Oncol 19:323, 1978

62. Caradonna, R, W Paladine, J Goldstein, et al Combination chemotherapy with high dose cis-diamminedichloroplatinum (II) (CDDP), methotrexate (MTX), and bleomycin (Bleo) for epidermoid carcinoma of the head and neck. Proceed Am Soc Clin Oncol 19:401, 1978

63. Elias, EG, PB Chretien, E Monnard, et al, Combination chemotherapy in advanced squamous cell carcinoma of the head and neck. Proceed Am Soc Clin Oncol 19:376, 1978

64. Wittes, R, K Heller, V Randolph, et al, Platinum-based chemotherapy as initial treatment in advanced head and neck cancer. Cancer Treat Rep (in press)

65. Goldsmith, MA, SK Carter, The integration of chemotherapy into a combined modality approach to cancer therapy. V. Squamous cell cancer of the head and neck. Cancer Treat Rev 2:137-158, 1975

66. Lustig, RA, PA DeMare, S Kramer, Adjuvant methotrexate in the radiotherapeutic management of advanced tumors of the head and neck. Cancer 37:2703-2708, 1976

CARCINOMA OF THE THYROID

Stephen C. Schimpff

Baltimore Cancer Research Program

of the Division of Cancer Treatment, NCI

at the University of Maryland Hospital

Baltimore, Maryland

EPIDEMIOLOGY

The incidence of thyroid carcinoma is low with about 8000 new cases per year in the United States. Worldwide, there is a wide variation among geographic areas (0.3 to 15 cases per 100,000 population per year) suggesting environmental influences to be predominant. The incidence among females is higher than for males, averaging about 3 to 1. The incidence rises steadily with age for males but rises rapidly in the third decade of life and then stabilizes for females. The overall sex differential is therefore due to these differences in rates among young adults. Since about 1940 there has been a trend toward a nearly three-fold increased incidence, principally among young adults. It is quite possible that this rising incidence is related to neck irradiation previously administered for benign conditions (1,2).

PATHOLOGY

Thyroid carcinomas are divided into those arising from the follicular or parafollicular (C-cells) epithelium (3). Those arising from the follicular epithelium may be differentiated (papillary, follicular) or undifferentiated anaplastic carcinoma whereas the parafollicular epithelial carcinomas are usually moderately well differentiated (medullary).

Designation as follicular carcinoma indicates that only follicular elements have been identified whereas tumors that are pure papillary or a mixture of papillary plus follicular elements are placed into the papillary carcinoma group. As a result, approximately 60% of thyroid carcinomas are classified as papillary and 20% are follicular, but if one reclassifies tumors based on the predominant histologic pattern, then the two types will be found in about equal frequency. In addition, careful review of multiple sections often shows evidence of the follicular pattern in one area and a papillary pattern elsewhere (4).

Papillary-Follicular

In the "pure" papillary form, there is very indolent growth with initial spread to the regional nodes, whereas the "pure" follicular carcinomas are more likely to show early blood vessel invasion with spread via blood borne metastases to bone and lung and, more rarely, to the regional nodes. There is a small proportion of follicular carcinomas that are well encapsulated and only rarely show vascular invasion; these may be hard to differentiate from the benign hypercellular fetal adenoma. Microscopic occult papillary carcinoma of the thyroid is not uncommon when thyroids removed at autopsy are subjected to multiple sectioning and careful evaluation (5). Similarly, if a total thyroidectomy is performed for a patient with a unilateral thyroid carcinoma, it is not uncommon to find a microscopic focus of disease in the contralateral lobe. Nevertheless, the prognosis for treated well differentiated carcinoma of the thyroid is excellent.

Anaplastic

The anaplastic tumors, unlike the papillary and follicular carcinomas, usually exhibit rapid growth. About 5% of all thyroid carcinomas are undifferentiated carcinomas with most being of the anaplastic type. These arise from differentiated tumors, rapidly destroy the capsule and extend widely into normal thyroid and surrounding tissues. Vascular invasion and lymphatic invasion is consistently observed with rapid spread by both the lymphatic and hematogenous routes. As a result, these tumors are usually very extensive at the time of initial diagnosis. The prognosis is dismal with death occurring in a few months.

Medullary

The tumors arising from the parafollicular or C-cells are the medullary carcinomas of the thyroid and represent about 5% of all thyroid cancers. This tumor is unique in its humoral properties, its occasional familial inheritance and its propensity to occur with other endocrine tumors. It is moderately well differentiated with a growth potential for spread intermediately between the papillary-follicular and the anaplastic carcinomas (6-8).

Metastases to Thyroid

Metastases to the thyroid are common with any widespread malignancy but the tumors which most commonly metastasize to the thyroid are hypernephroma, and carcinomas of the larynx, esophagus, lung and rectum.

Prognostic Factors

The WHO classification of thyroid carcinoma is of prognostic value. In a series of 964 cases of thyroid cancer followed for 5-30 years, the percent of patients who had died was 11% with papillary carcinoma, 24% with follicular carcinoma, 50% with medullary carcinoma, and 90% with undifferentiated carcinomas (9). Follicular tumors are more frequent in middle and older individuals and, with their blood borne metastatic potential, it is perhaps not surprising that prognosis is worse for follicular than for papillary carcinomas. Since papillary carcinomas metastasize initially to local nodes, the opportunity for surgical cure is greater. Large differentiated tumors have a poorer prognosis than small ones, but extension through the thyroid capsule substantially worsens survival. In one series, for example, a small tumor entirely confined to the thyroid was associated with only 9% mortality compared to 16% if the tumor were greater than 4 cm. The mortality increased to 39% when there was any extraglandular tumor (9). For unclear reasons, age has a marked prognostic effect with the highest survival being in the youngest and the lowest survival being in the oldest (10). To summarize, considerable prognostic information can be derived for a patient with recently identified thyroid carcinoma by considering the histologic type, tumor size, the presence or absence of capsular or angioinvasion, multiple foci, nodal or distant metastases, plus the patient's age.

PATHOGENESIS

Chronic Stimulation

Chronic stimulation of the thyroid by thyroid stimulating hormone (TSH) may occasionally induce thyroid carcinoma in some animal species. Likewise, irradiation in doses sufficient to damage but not destroy the gland may induce occasional tumors. In the rat, a combination of low dose irradiation plus chronic TSH stimulation (induced by methylthiouracil) will lead to carcinoma in most animals within about one year (11). Similarly, a chemical carcinogen plus TSH stimulation in rats will increase the incidence and shorten the latency period. The mechanism whereby physical or chemical carcinogens plus TSH stimulation affects neoplasia is not known but a reasonable hypothesis is that the carcinogen induces a permanent, nonreversible alteration in the thyroid epithelial cell, but cancer is not expressed in most cases because the mitotic activity of thyroid tissue is low. The mechanism for tumor induction is presumably that, because TSH stimulates mitosis, there is an increased likelihood that the irradiation altered cells will divide and proceed to tumor development. Although elevated TSH levels are an important co-factor in the development of thyroid carcinoma in the rat following moderate dose irradiation, most humans found to have thyroid carcinoma do not have a concomitant elevation of TSH at the time of diagnosis (12). It is possible that there are other substances with TSH activity slightly different from the recognized human TSH which may be capable of stimulating the thyroid gland and acting as a co-factor toward thyroid carcinoma when accompanied by prior irradiation. Some patients with thyroid carcinoma have been found to have a biologically active TSH which is reactive in the radioimmunoassay for bovine but not human TSH (13).

The only recognized cause of thyroid cancer in humans is irradiation. The relative risk increased by a factor of 2.5 in individuals with excess alcohol consumption, perhaps by inducing a state of TSH excess (14). The higher incidence of carcinoma at younger ages for females compared to males suggests an additional hormonal feature, perhaps a pituitary hormone or an HCG-like hormone with some potential to activate TSH binding sites.

Irradiation

Among the survivors of Hiroshima and Nagasaki, a 5 to 9.4 increase in the relative risk for developing clinically evident thyroid carcinoma has been detected for those who received 50 or more rads (15). A higher level of irradiation did not correlate with a higher relative risk, but cases were detected among those who received lower irradiation doses. The 74 detected tumors have been predominately papillary forms with follicular elements being uncommon. No case of anaplastic or medullary carcinoma has occurred. Unlike acute leukemia which reached a peak incidence by 1951 and has been declining since, the peak incidence for irradiation-related thyroid carcinoma has probably not yet been obtained, indicating a very prolonged latency period. As in the general population, the overall risk has been higher for women than for men.

In 1954, residents of several atolls in the Marshall Islands were exposed to an average of 335 rads of thyroid-seeking nucleides of iodine as a result of radioactive fallout from thermonuclear bomb testing over Bikini (16). As of 1976, 40 of 243 exposed Marshallese (16.5%) had developed thyroid nodules. The occurrence of nodules has been more common in children than adults, females than males, and there appears to be a dose-response relationship. Among these 40 have been seven documented cases of thyroid cancer with a latency period of 11 to 22 years.

The risk of developing thyroid adenomas or carcinomas following low dose radiation therapy was not generally appreciated until recently. There are large numbers of Americans who were treated with irradiation for enlarged thymus, hypertrophied tonsils or adenoids, adolescent acne, tinea capitis, cervical adenitis, pertussis or keloids of the upper torso in the period 1910-1950. The thyroid had been considered relatively radioresistant and the usual dose of irradiation utilized for these conditions was low. However, in 1950, Duffy and Fitzgerald (17) observed that among children with differentiated thyroid carcinoma, 36% had prior irradiation to the neck area; a similar report came from Clark (18) in 1955. Multiple reports since that time have documented a very substantial risk of developing benign or malignant thyroid tumors ten or more years after childhood neck irradiation. For example, in an evaluation of 100 consecutive adults with a history of irradiation to the neck during childhood, 26 were found to have an abnormality by thyroid palpation (19). Eight of those 15 who had surgery had benign thyroid lesions and 7 had carcinomas. Among those 7 otherwise asymptomatic individuals found to have cancer, 5 already had invasive or locally disseminated disease. Thus, the incidence of thyroid carcinoma in this group is at least 7%. In another survey in which 1560 individuals with a history of childhood neck irradiation were screened with physical examination and ^{99m}Te scanning, 20% were found to have abnormalities sufficient to recommend surgery (20). Similar to the earlier study, this evaluation found a 7% incidence of detected carcinoma in the total population screened and a 33% incidence of cancer among those with clinically detectable lesions. These data interpreted in light of the known extensive use of irradiation for multiple benign conditions in past years indicates that a very large population exists who are at high risk for developing thyroid carcinoma. It is therefore imperative that all patients be questioned about the possibility of prior neck irradiation. Those with a positive response should have yearly evaluations including careful neck palpation and possibly ^{123}I or ^{99m}Te scans to detect lesions as early as possible. Any recognized abnormalities should prompt open surgical biopsy with careful extensive review of pathological sections (21).

TREATMENT OF WELL DIFFERENTIATED THYROID CARCINOMAS

Treatment alternatives

The treatment of the well differentiated thyroid carcinomas is controversial. The major issues are whether a careful removal of all apparent tumor including neck metastases followed by thyroid hormone suppression of TSH is sufficient for most patients with papillary carcinoma or whether a majority of patients should also be treated postoperatively with radioactive iodine. Among the reasons for the lack of agreement on the proper approach to these patients are the total absence of satisfactory controlled trials, a generally excellent prognosis so that only evaluations comparing many patients will be likely to show differences in end results and inadequate followup periods for most reports because of the indolent growth patterns.

With recurrence rates as low as they are for surgery followed with thyroid hormone even including lobectomy with limited node removal, one can question whether further aggressive measures should be taken. The excellent longterm survival of patients with papillary carcinoma following surgery may be misleading however. Survival need not represent disease-free survival and, since follow-up of large numbers of patients over long periods has rarely been achieved, ultimate prognosis especially for young individuals is not entirely clear. Multiple evaluations do note recurrences with perhaps 20-30% of patients having recurrences within 15-20 years. This represents a high rate of disease return and indicates the need for improved therapy.

Surgery versus Surgery + RAI

In 1970, Varma et al (22) reported a comparison between the survival of 263 patients treated with surgery plus radioactive iodine (RAI) from 1947 to 1964 and 50 patients treated with surgery alone from 1933 to 1947. Those with papillary carcinoma had a 37% death rate in the control group and 9% in the RAI group. Survival was less satisfactory for follicular carcinoma with death rates of 45% and 19% for control and RAI groups respectively. Survival for all RAI treated patients depended upon adequacy of ^{131}I uptake ablation. Among 229 patients with normal scans after ^{131}I, the death rate was 3% but rose to 59% for the 34 patients with persistent uptake after the last ^{131}I dose. These differences pertained for both papillary and follicular histology.

Krishnamurthy and Blahd (23) gave RAI after completion of total or subtotal thyroidectomy and excision of involved cervical lymph nodes to 54 patients. A dose of 75-150 mCi was administered about six weeks postoperatively following three daily injections of 10 units of bovine TSH. Patients were retreated every six months until scans indicated total uptake ablation. All patients received thyroid hormone replacement. The mean cumulative ablative dose was 163.4 mCi (range 75-630) but was higher (average 195 mCi) for those with initial evidence of metastases. None of the 44 patients with papillary or follicular carcinoma who had total ablation died. Recurrences, based on the development of scan abnormalities, occurred in 10 of these 44 patients, but were more common in those with initial metastases (56%) than those without (25%) metastases. Not only did follicular and mixed papillary-follicular carcinomas take up ^{131}I, but in this series all 24 patients with papillary carcinoma had uptake and 23 of 24 had total ablation with RAI. There were also a few undifferentiated (2) and Hurthle cell (2) tumors treated, none of which showed ablation with all four patients dying of thyroid cancer.

In another series studying only papillary and papillary-follicular carcinoma, Mazzaferri et al (24) evaluated the results obtained among 576 individuals treated with or without RAI. Follow-up was from 6 months to 30 years and averaged 7 years. The recurrence rate and the mortality rate were significantly lower for patients who received ^{131}I plus thyroid hormone than for those who received postoperative thyroid hormone alone, external irradiation or no adjunctive therapy. Only three (3%) of those (114) treated with RAI and thyroid hormone had a recurrence whereas there was a four-fold higher recurrence rate (45 of 414 or 11%) for those who received postoperative thyroid hormone and there was a 40% (12 of 30) recurrence rate among those patients who received no postoperative thyroid hormones. As to deaths due to thyroid cancer, none of those receiving RAI plus thyroid hormone or those receiving thyroid hormone alone died but 4 or 13% of those with no postoperative therapy died. Among 310 patients with near or total thyroidectomy, the recurrence rate was only 2% (2 of 94) if RAI was administered compared to 8% (17 of 204) if RAI was not given. For patients with limited thyroid surgery and no RAI, the addition of thyroid hormone postoperatively reduced recurrences to 15% (12 of 78) compared to 62% (8 of 13) when no thyroid hormone was given. The following factors were of independent significance with regard to recurrences: 1) Age - younger patients had a higher recurrence rate despite a lower death rate, 2) Primary Lesion Size - the larger the primary lesion, the greater the risk of recurrence, 3) Extent of Local Invasion - invasion through the thyroid capsule (irrespective of cervical node metastases which had no prognostic effect) was associated with more recurrences than those without local tumor extension, 4) Adjunctive Medical Therapy - as discussed above, the addition of thyroid hormone, RAI or both reduced recurrences substantially.

Despite the data favoring postoperative radioactive iodine ablation therapy, there is no data indicating whether it is better to administer RAI to everyone immediately or to wait and give RAI only should there be a recurrence. Since one can make some reasonable estimation of prognosis at the time of initial evaluation, it would seem reasonable to utilize RAI for those patients with a large tumor, blood vessel or capsular invasion, node involvement or substantial follicular elements. In others, surgery alone plus lifelong TSH suppression with thyroid hormone may be sufficient. All patients require close follow-up since recurrences may not be apparent for 10, 20 or more years.

CYTOTOXIC DRUG THERAPY

Not all differentiated tumors will incorporate ^{131}I so that other therapeutic modalities are indicated for some patients with extensive metastases not amenable to surgery. There is only limited data available on the effectiveness of cytotoxic agents for the treatment of thyroid carcinoma. In the review by Gottlieb et al (25) 55 courses of single or multiple agent chemotherapy were administered to 37 patients. Partial responses included 3 of 5 patients given adriamycin, one of 5 given methotrexate, and one of 3 given phenylaline mustard. There were no other responses including none among those who received 5-fluorouracil, actinomycin D, cyclophosphamide or various combinations. The results with adriamycin prompted further evaluation of that drug in a prospective trial. Of 22 treated patients, 3 achieved a complete remission and 4 had a partial remission. These responses were notable in that they occurred in patients with differentiated thyroid cancer, especially among those with oxyphilic (Hurthle cell) elements but responses were nil in patients with anaplastic carcinoma. Pulmonary and osseous metastasis responded better than other sites. Bleomycin was used for 21 patients, most with well differentiated tumors, by Haroda et al (26) who noted softening or shrinkage of 9 of 11 primary tumor sites and 25 of the 29 involved nodes which were evaluated. Obviously, further drug studies are necessary to establish active agents and combinations.

MEDULLARY CARCINOMA OF THE THYROID

Medullary carcinoma was first described in 1959 (27) and, although representing less than 5% of all thyroid cancers, has been extensively studied because of its unusual characteristics. Although most of these tumors arise spontaneously, the familial form with autosomal dominant inheritance is part of the multiple endocrine adenomatosis syndrome, type II (Sipple's syndrome) (6,7,8).

Sipple's Syndrome

This syndrome has three major components: medullary carcinoma of the thyroid, pheochromocytoma and parathyroid hyperplasia (28). An individual patient may have any one, two or all three components. The thyroid and the adrenal medullary tumors are usually multicentric and frequently bilateral.

Calcitonin is characteristically secreted by the medullary carcinoma of the thyroid (29,30) but a substance similar or perhaps identical to calcitonin has been isolated from the adrenal medulla. Conversely, an adrenomedullary enzyme, decarboxylase, can occasionally be isolated from medullary thyroid carcinoma tissue (7). Even in patients who do not have a pheochromocytoma, close inspection of the adrenal medulla will show hyperplasia in nearly all individuals. Similarly, close sectioning of an involved resected thyroid will show C-cell hyperplasia in many areas irrespective of the specific location of one or more medullary carcinomas. The parathyroids usually do not show adenoma formation but rather hyperplasia. Thus, each of the three affected organs are involved with a process of hyperplasia which in two of the three (thyroid and adrenal medulla) frequently results in adenoma or carcinoma formation. It has been suggested that the parathyroid hyperplasia is compensation for the effect of the calcitonin produced by the medullary carcinoma of the thyroid, but some family members with this syndrome have been found to have elevated serum parathormone levels prior to the initial elevation of calcitonin indicating that the parathyroid abnormality is probably part of the primary genetic defect and not simply a secondary response.

Hormone Abnormalities in Medullary Carcinoma

The hormones secreted by the medullary carcinoma of the thyroid include calcitonin and histaminase in all patients plus ACTH, prostaglandins and serotonin in many (6). Calcitonin lowers serum calcium but parathyroid hyperplasia or adenoma formation with parathormone secretion will maintain a normal serum calcium level. Basal serum calcitonin levels are usually elevated irrespective of tumor size. The remaining patients will have an abnormal elevation of calcitonin following a four hour calcium infusion test. Histaminase activity is always elevated in resected tumor tissue but may not be elevated in the serum of patients with localized tumor (7). Histaminase is frequently elevated, however, in the serum of patients with metastatic disease and follow-up levels of serum histaminase postoperatively may prove to be a good marker for the presence or absence of residual disease (7). Prostaglandins, serotonin, or both may be responsible for the watery diarrhea which occurs in some of these patients. Finally, the ectopic ACTH syndrome may rarely occur in association with this tumor (7).

Patterns of Presentation

Medullary carcinoma of the thyroid, unlike the papillary-follicular carcinomas, occurs in either sex with approximately equal frequency and occurs over a wide age range. The majority of tumors are probably spontaneous in origin but careful family studies are required for all patients to rule out the possibility of an autosomal dominant transmitted disease. Some individuals will have mucosal neuromata, especially of the oral mucosa. This constellation of neuromata and medullary carcinoma suggests the potential for bilateral pheochromocytoma. A loose watery diarrhea occurs in about one-third of patients and may be associated with other symptoms and signs suggesting a carcinoid syndrome.

Medullary carcinoma is usually multicentric in origin and tends to locally invade early in its development, frequently when the tumor is much smaller than that which is palpable. It progresses first to local lymph nodes, including early dissemination to the mediastinum, and concurrently may progress by hematogenous dissemination to lung and bone (6). Both primary and metastatic lesions may calcify and be radiologically demonstrable (6,7). Medullary carcinoma of the thyroid is usually described as being of intermediate aggressiveness when scaled between the differentiated carcinomas and the anaplastic carcinomas of the thyroid. Individual tumors, however, can have widely varying degrees of growth potential.

Therapy of Medullary Carcinoma

Because of the frequent bilateral involvement, early regional lymph node involvement and lung and bone involvement, an early aggressive surgical approach is indicated. In the absence of known metastatic disease, a total thyroidectomy is indicated. Lobectomy or less than total thyroidectomy has a high likelihood of leaving behind another focus of tumor. In addition, there should be dissection of lymph nodes extending substernally into the mediastinum as far as possible. In one study of the familial disease by Melvin (31), about 50% of patients had lymph node involvement of the neck when the primary thyroid tumor was still less than 1 mm. in size. It has not been demonstrated, however, whether radical neck dissection is of any benefit.

The tumor is not TSH responsive and hence suppressive therapy with thyroid hormone should not be expected to be beneficial. Likewise, ^{131}I therapy will not be useful for either local or metastatic disease. Chemotherapy has also not been of much value for medullary carcinoma of the thyroid, although adriamycin has produced occasional responses.

Spontaneous medullary carcinoma is usually first detected as a thyroid nodule followed by diagnosis at frozen section during open surgical biopsy. The surgeon should then complete a total thyroidectomy and a careful lymph node dissection. Since, at this point, it will not be known if the patient has the familial syndrome, the parathyroid should be carefully evaluated with removal of adenomatous tissue. Postoperatively, there should be a search for pheochromocytoma.

Screening for Medullary Carcinoma

Utilization of radioimmunoassay for detection of calcitonin in family members of afflicted patients has made screening for medullary carcinoma of the thyroid a relatively simple procedure. In the initial study by Melvin et al., (30) 83 members of a family in whom medullary thyroid carcinoma had been proven in 7 were studied. Calcitonin was obtained in the basal state and following a four hour calcium infusion. Medullary thyroid carcinoma was predicted in 12 of these 83 tested individuals and, at subsequent surgery, all 12 were proven to have disease. Thus, a positive assay correlates closely with the presence of disease. Since then it has been shown that repeated testing of individuals on a yearly basis will give early evidence of the present of this tumor with a high degree of accuracy. Individuals whose calcitonin assay converts from negative to positive should be subjected to total thyroidectomy. In their most recent follow-up (32), an additional 21 individuals from this single pedigree, now numbering 107, have converted from normal to abnormal secretory responses. Surgery revealed C-cell hyperplasia in 20, plus carcinoma in eight. Unlike the original 12 patients, none of those eight individuals with recent conversion had local metastases, the tumor tended to be smaller and all eight were unilateral. In view of these findings, it is not surprising that the age of detection was younger (mean age of 15 years) in this group than in the previous twelve (mean age 36 years) (32).

Before total thyroidectomy, however, the patient should also be screened for the possibility of pheochromocytoma. The incidence of pheochromocytoma is high and the anesthesia risks require that this tumor be managed prior to removal of the medullary carcinoma of the thyroid. Pheochromocytomas in this population almost always occur in the adrenals but frequently are bilateral. As noted above, careful sectioning of adrenals from these patients even in the absence of an overt pheochromocytoma will usually show adrenal medullary hyperplasia.

To summarize, medullary carcinoma of the thyroid is rare and represents less than five percent of all thyroid tumors. Although usually sporadic in occurrence, it can be part of a familial disease associated with pheochromocytoma and parathyroid adenoma. It is important to recognize that this is an aggressive tumor which metastasizes both locally and distantly in its early stages, that it is usually bilateral and multicentric and therefore, the initial surgical approach should be aggressive including total thyroidectomy with careful removal of involved neck nodes. The advent of the radioimmunoassay for calcitonin will establish the diagnosis preoperatively and, more importantly, serves as an excellent screening device for families with the multiple endocrine adenomatosis syndrome.

SUMMARY

Thyroid carcinoma is rare but of increasing public health importance because of the widespread use of neck irradiation for benign conditions in years past. The latency period is 10, 20 or more years with, currently, about 7% having detectable cancer. Most irradiation-related carcinomas are papillary or papillary-follicular types.

Treatment of the differentiated carcinomas includes careful resection followed by lifelong TSH suppression with thyroid hormone. Patients with large tumors, angioinvasion, capsular invasion, local or distant metastases probably should be treated with radioactive iodine ablation of all remaining iodine concentrating tissue following total or near total thyroidectomy. Adjunctive TSH suppression for life is also indicated. Follow-up must be for life with yearly evaluations.

Recurrent tumors should be treated with radioactive iodine or, perhaps, cytotoxic agents such as adriamycin. Anaplastic tumors require external beam irradiation; surgery, radioactive iodine, thyroid hormone and adriamycin are usually of little or no value.

Medullary carcinoma of the thyroid arises from the parafollicular (C-cells) epithelium. It is usually spontaneous in occurrence and unicentric. However, some families have the autosomal dominant multiple endocrine adenomatosis syndrome II which includes medullary carcinoma of the thyroid, pheochromocytoma and parathyroid hyperplasia. Family members should have calcitonin assays, basal and after calcium infusion, performed at least yearly to detect medullary thyroid carcinoma while it is still small and localized to the thyroid.

REFERENCES

1. Schottenfeld, D and S Gershman, Epidemiology of thyroid cancer. Cancer 28:66-86, 1978

2. Sancho-Garnier, H, Epidemiology of thyroid cancer. Ann Radiol 20:715-721, 1977

3. Histological typing of thyroid tumours, International Histological Classification of Tumours, No. II, World Health Organization, Geneva, 1974

4. Franssila, KO, Is the differentiation between papillary and follicualar thyroid carcinoma valid? Cancer 32:853-864, 1973

5. Mortensen, JD, WA Bennett, and LB Woolner, Incidence of carcinoma in thyroid glands removed at 1,000 consecutive routine necropsies. Surg Forum 5:659-663, 1954

6. Hill, CS, Jr, ML Ibanez, NA Samaan, et al, Medullary (solid) carcinoma of the thyroid gland: An analysis of the M.D. Anderson Hospital experience with patients with tumor, its special features, and its histogenesis. Medicine 52:141-171, 1973

7. Baylin, SB, Medullary carcinoma of the thyroid gland: Use of biochemical parameters in detection and surgical management of the tumor. Surg Clin No Amer 54:309-323, 1974

8. Sizemore, GW, JA Carney, and H Heath, III, Epidemiology of medullary carcinoma of the thyroid gland: A 5-year experience (1971-1976). Surg Clin No Amer 57:633-645, 1977

9. Cady, B, CE Sedwick, WA Meissner, et al, Changing clinical, pathologic treatment and survival patterns in differentiated thyroid carcinoma. Ann Surg 184:541-552, 1976

10. Halnan, KE, Influence of age and sex on incidence and prognosis of thyroid cancer. Three hundred forty-four cases followed for ten years. Cancer 19:1534-1536, 1966

11. Doniach, I, The effect of radioactive iodine alone and in combination with methylthiouracil and acetylaminofluorene upon tumor production in the rat's thyroid gland. Brit J Cancer 4:223-234, 1950

12. LeMarchand-Beraud, T, BR Scazziga, C Berthier, et al, Pituitary regulation and T_3 nuclear binding in thyroid carcinoma. Ann Radiol 20:731-734, 1977

13. LeMarchand-Beraud, T, M Griessen, and BR Scazziga, Comparison of bovine and human TSH radioimmunoassay for human plasma TSH determination and correlation with bioassay. In: Further Advances in Thyroid Research, Fellinger, K and R Hofer (eds), Wien, Verlag de Wierner Medizinischen Akademie, 1971

14. Williams, RR, Breast and thyroid cancer and malignant melanoma promoted by alcohol induced pituitary secretion of prolactin, TSH, MSH. Lancet i:996-999, 1976

15. Parker, LN, JL Belsky, T Yamamoto, et al, Thyroid carcinoma after exposure to atomic radiation. A continuing survey of a fixed population, Hiroshima and Nagasaki, 1958-1971. Ann Intern Med 80:600-604, 1974

16. Conard, RA, Summary of thyroid findings in Marshallese 22 years after exposure to radioactive fallout. In: Radiation-Associated Thyroid Carcinoma. DeGroot, LJ (ed), New York, Grune and Stratton, pp 241-257, 1977

17. Duffy, BJ, Jr. and PJ Fitzgerald, Cancer of the thyroid in children: A report of 28 cases. J Clin Endocrinol 10:1296-1308, 1950

18. Clark, DE, Association of irradiation with cancer of the thyroid in children and adolescents. JAMA 159:1007-1009, 1955

19. Refetoff, S, J. Harrison, J, BT Karanfilski, et al, Continuing occurrence of thyroid carcinoma after irradiation to the neck in infancy and childhood. New Engl J Med 292:171-175, 1975

20. Favus, MJ, AB Schneider, MD Stachura, et al, Thyroid cancer occurring as late consequence of head and neck irradiation. New Engl J Med 294:1019-1025, 1976

21. National Cancer Institute - Division of Cancer Control and Rehabilitation, Irradiation-related thyroid cancer. U.S. Department of Health, Education and Welfare, DHEW Publication No. (NIH) 77-1120.

22. Varma, VM, WH Beierwaltes, MM Nofal, et al, Treatment of thyroid cancer: Death rates after surgery and after surgery followed by sodium iodide I 131. JAMA 214:1437-1442, 1970

23. Krishnamurthy, GT and WH Blahd, Radioiodine I-131 therapy in the management of thyroid cancer: A prospective study. Cancer 40:195-202, 1977

24. Mazzaferri, EL, RL Young, JE Oertel, et al, Papillary thyroid carcinoma: The impact of therapy in 576 patients. Medicine 56:171-196, 1977

25. Gottlieb, JA, CS Hill, and JR Stratton, Adriamycin (NSC-123127) therapy in thyroid carcinoma. Cancer Chemother Rep 6:283-296, 1975

26. Harada, T, Y Nishikawa, T Suzuki,et al, Bleomycin treatment for cancer of the thyroid. Amer J Surg 122:53-57, 1971

27. Hazard, JB, WA Hawk, and G Crile, Jr, Medullary (solid) carcinoma of the thyroid gland. J Clin Endocrin 19:152-161, 1959

28. Sipple, JH, The association of pheochromocytoma with carcinoma of the thyroid gland. Amer J Med 31:163-166, 1961

29. Tashjian, AH, Jr and KEW Melvin, Medullary carcinoma of the thyroid gland: Studies of thyrocalcitonin in plasma and tumor extracts. New Engl J Med 279:279-283, 1968

30. Tashjian, AH, Jr, BG Howland, KEW Melvin, et al, Immunoassay of human calcitonin. Clinical measurement, relation to serum calcium and studies in patients with medullary carcinoma. New Engl J Med 283:890-895, 1970

31. Melvin, KEW, HH Miller, and AH Tashjian, Jr, Early diagnosis of medullary carcinoma of the thyroid gland by means of calcitonin assay. New Engl J Med 285:1115-1120, 1971

32. Graze, K, IJ Spiler, AH, Tashjian, Jr, et al, Natural history of familial medullary thyroid carcinoma. Effect of a program for early diagnosis. New Engl J Med 299:980-985, 1978

COMPUTED TOMOGRAPHY IN THE EVALUATION OF ABDOMINAL MALIGNANCY

David H. Stephens, M.D. and Patrick F. Sheedy, II, M.D.
Department of Diagnostic Radiology
Mayo Clinic
Rochester, Minnesota

INTRODUCTION

Throughout the four years that computed tomography (CT) has been capable of abdominal examination, a major application of the method has been the evaluation of patients known or suspected to have abdominal malignancy (1-8). CT has been especially effective in the detection of neoplasms located in sites that are least accessible to conventional radiography -- in the solid organs of the abdomen and in the retroperitoneal space. In addition to permitting the initial detection of tumors, CT provides clinically useful information about their size, extent, and effect on neighboring structures. The precise localizing ability of CT has led to its increased utilization in percutaneous aspiration biopsy of abdominal masses (9, 10) and in radiation treatment planning (11,12). Particularly relevant to medical oncology is the ability of CT to detect recurrence of certain tumors in post-operative patients and to permit accurate assessment of tumor response in patients who undergo non-surgical therapy.

Although still considered to be in its early stages of development, CT has undergone rapid technologic advancement since its introduction. Images that were produced by early scanners already appear primitive by current standards. Among the many improvements found in newer machines is the ability to perform a scan in a few seconds, thereby eliminating the artifactual problems caused by respiratory and peristaltic motion. The latest instruments are capable of computer reconstructions in the sagittal and coronal planes as well as producing cross-sectional displays of anatomy.

CLINICAL APPLICATIONS

For convenience, the clinical applications of abdominal CT will be discussed in the customary manner, organ by organ. This approach, however, tends to obscure one of the major advantages of abdominal CT scanning: the information provided is not limited to a single organ or system (Figure 1). Thus, an examination that is directed primarily at one organ may reveal related or unexpected abnormalities at other sites.

104

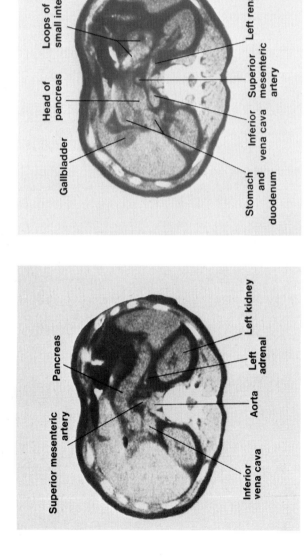

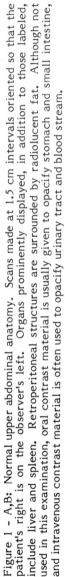

Figure 1 - A,B: Normal upper abdominal anatomy. Scans made at 1.5 cm intervals oriented so that the patient's right is on the observer's left. Organs prominently displayed, in addition to those labeled, include liver and spleen. Retroperitoneal structures are surrounded by radiolucent fat. Although not used in this examination, oral contrast material is usually given to opacify stomach and small intestine, and intravenous contrast material is often used to opacify urinary tract and blood stream.

(From Sheedy, PF, II, DH Stephens, RR Hattery, RL MacCarty, B Williamson, Jr. Radiol Clin N Amer 15:349, 1977 with permission)

Liver and Biliary Tree

CT may be used either as the initial method to detect hepatic neoplasms or as a complementary method to confirm the presence or clarify the nature of a lesion detected by another modality (13-19). Radionuclide liver scanning, because it is highly sensitive, relatively inexpensive, and easily performed, remains the primary screening examination in most practices (16-18). The initial detection of hepatic metastases by CT often occurs on examinations that are requested to evaluate other abdominal organs, as the liver is included in most abdominal CT studies, whether or not it is the primary organ of interest (Figure 2). When surgical resection of a known hepatic tumor is being considered, CT, in conjunction with angiography, provides useful information regarding the precise location and extent of the lesion.

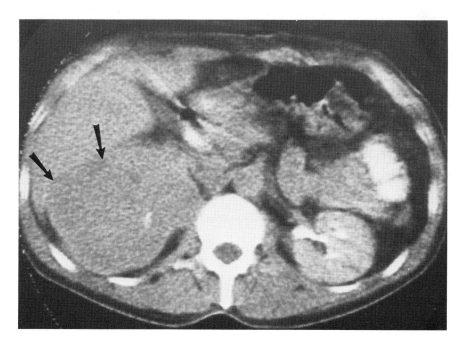

Figure 2A: Renal cell carcinoma with hepatic metastasis. Large soft tissue mass (arose) arises from the lateral aspect of the right kidney.

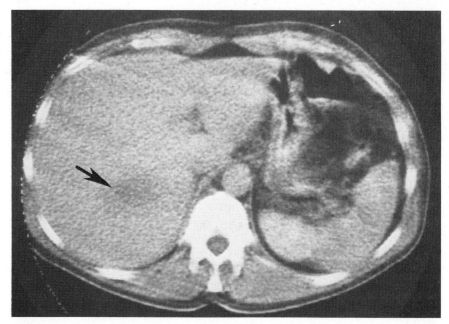

Figure 2B: Renal cell carcinoma with hepatic metastasis. Scan at higher level shows solitary metastatic tumor in the right lobe of the liver.

Masses within the liver are detectable when their radiographic densities differ appreciably from that of the adjacent normal hepatic parenchyma. Most neoplasms are of slightly diminished radiographic density relative to normal liver (Figures 2,3). Because of the variation in density among normal livers and among hepatic tumors, however, occasional tumors are of a density that is indistinguishable from normal parenchyma and therefore may escape detection. The use of intravenous contrast material sometimes permits detection of lesions that cannot be appreciated on unenhanced scans.

The differential diagnosis of hepatic masses by CT is based on differences in their radiographic densities and other characteristics. Solid tumors are readily distinguished from cysts and abscesses. Necrotic tumors may resemble abscesses, but the differentiation can usually be made with clinical correlation. Hepatomas and other primary liver neoplasms cannot be differentiated from metastases on the basis of density alone. Although multiple small tumors are likely to be metastatic, hepatomas may be multifocal; and, conversely, metastases may be solitary. In most cases of metastasis, however, the primary tumor is already known or suspected to be present.

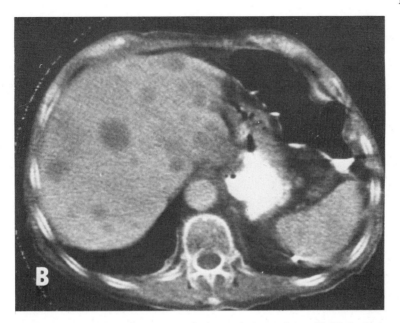

Figure 3: Liver metastases from carcinoma of the colon. Multiple lesions of diminished density are distributed throughout the liver. Note opacification of the stomach with contrast material.

(From MacCarty, RL, DH Stephens, RR Hattery, PF Sheedy, II. Radiol Clin N Amer 17:137, 1979 with permission)

Because of its ability to display dilated intrahepatic and extrahepatic bile ducts, CT is a highly accurate method to differentiate obstructive from non-obstructive jaundice (20). When the biliary obstruction is caused by a neoplasm, CT often shows the mass lesion as well as the dilated ducts.

Pancreas

Few challenges in radiology have been as perplexing as the diagnosis of pancreatic cancer. Until the development of modern imaging techniques, the pancreas itself could not be visualized, and radiologic detection of pancreatic tumors was dependent for the most part on secondary evidence of the disease. On properly performed CT examinations, the entire pancreas can be displayed almost routinely (Figure 1). In most cases of pancreatic cancer, the tumor can now be detected with little compromise of the patient's safety or comfort.

Most pancreatic carcinomas are of the same radiographic density as the normal pancreas. Therefore, in order for a solid tumor of the pancreas to be detected by CT, the mass must either be large enough to alter the contour of the pancreas or extend beyond the confines of the gland (Figure 4).

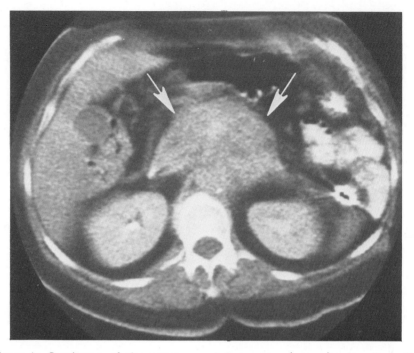

Figure 4: Carcinoma of the pancreas. A large mass (arrows) arises from the body of the pancreas and obliterates the retropancreatic fat in front of the aorta.

Enlargement of the pancreatic image usually takes the form of a focal mass. Neoplastic infiltration into the adjacent tissues is often evident. Zones of diminished density within a tumor may result from tissue necrosis.

Dilatation of biliary or pancreatic ducts are prominent secondary features in many patients with cancer of the head of the pancreas. A significant proportion of patients with carcinoma of the pancreatic head, however, have obvious masses without clinical jaundice or CT evidence of ductal obstruction. Other common secondary findings in patients with pancreatic carcinoma include metastases involving the liver or nearby lymph nodes.

Currently available contrast materials are of limited value in the detection of pancreatic carcinoma. Some highly vascular islet cell tumors become opacified with intravenous contrast material, and pancreatic cysts and dilated ducts may be shown more distinctly after contrast enhancements of the surrounding parenchyma.

All recent reports of experiences using modern CT equipment indicate CT to be an accurate method to diagnose pancreatic cancer among symptomatic patients (21-26). Although tumors that remain confined to the pancreas and are too small to distort its contour are not likely to be detected, it appears that very few persons with such early tumors are symptomatic enough to seek medical attention.

Even among symptomatic patients, there have been both false negative and false positive CT diagnoses, though accuracy has improved with technological improvements and with increased interpreter experience. A cause of false positive diagnosis of pancreatic cancer is the presence of another mass involving or immediately adjacent to the pancreas. Pancreatitis occasionally causes focal enlargement of the gland that is indistinguishable from tumor, and neoplasms arising from adjacent tissues can blend imperceptibly with the pancreatic image. Occasional pancreatic CT examinations produce indeterminate results, either because the organ is not satisfactorily imaged or because the findings are not definitive. In those cases, information provided by other diagnostic examinations is essential.

Although CT has become established as an accurate and convenient method to diagnose or exclude pancreatic cancer, there is little evidence that the method is likely to alter the distressingly poor prognosis in this condition. By the time they come to clinical attention, most carcinomas of the pancreas are beyond the stage at which a cure is possible. However, even though most pancreatic cancers that are discovered will not be resectable, CT can usually provide the diagnosis and reveal the extent of the disease early in the work-up and thereby obviate the need for more complex, more invasive, and often less informative procedures. When a tumor is shown to be obviously unresectable, percutaneous aspiration biopsy may circumvent laparotomy. Perhaps of more practical significance than the detection of pancreatic cancer is its exclusion. The demonstration of a normal pancreas is itself an important finding, as in most cases attention can then be directed toward another cause of the patient's symptoms.

Adrenal Glands

CT is a rapid and reliable method to evaluate the morphology of the adrenal glands (27-30). With modern CT equipment, the adrenals can be visualized in almost all adults. CT has become our preferred method to evaluate the adrenal glands in most patients who have clinical, biochemical or radiographic evidence of adrenal neoplasms. Because of the small size of normal adrenal glands, very small tumors, such as aldosterone secreting adenomas, can often be detected. Most malignant neoplasms are considerably larger and are readily discovered. Metastatic tumors of the adrenal glands are occasional unexpected findings in patients being evaluated for other primary neoplasms.

Kidneys

CT joins other diagnostic imaging procedures as a highly reliable, though not infallible, method to detect renal neoplasms and differentiate them from benign cysts (31-34). The characteristics of renal masses are similar to those demonstrated by ultrasonography, angiography and nephrotomography. A cyst usually appears as a sharply marginated, homogenous, rounded structure with a density near that of water; whereas a tumor usually has an indistinct interface with the renal parenchyma, nonhomogeneous density, and a thick irregular wall (Figure 2A). The density of a tumor increases after intravenous administration of contrast material, while the density of a cyst remains essentially unchanged. In cases of renal carcinoma, CT may demonstrate extrarenal extention of the tumor or distant metastases.

In our practice, CT has been particularly useful to evaluate patients suspected to have recurrent tumor following nephrectomy for renal carcinoma (Figure 5).

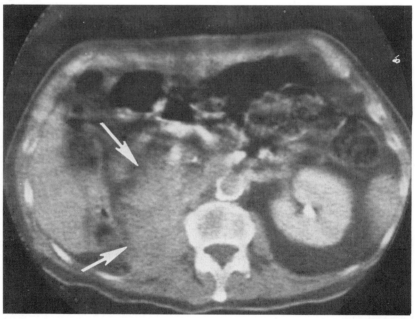

Figure 5: Recurrent renal carcinoma. Scan made nine months after right nephrectomy for renal cell carcinoma shows an extensive recurrent tumor (arrows) in the right renal bed.

Abdominal Lymphadenopathy

In order to be detected by CT, diseased abdominal lymph nodes must be appreciably enlarged. In most cases of retroperitoneal lymphoma, and in many cases of metastatic lymphadenopathy, the involved nodes are readily detected. Nodal enlargement is easiest to recognize when it involves the para-aortic nodes, which are normally well outlined by intraabdominal redundant fat. Lymphadenopathy may also be detected within the mesentery and abdominal locations. The CT appearance of malignant retroperitoneal lymphadenopathy varies from a small number of discrete enlarged nodes to a more conglomerate group of contiguous nodes to a large homogeneous confluent mass of nodes that obliterate the margins of the aorta and vena cava. Although the CT appearance does not allow differentiation between benign and malignant nodal enlargement, this limitation is seldom a problem in evaluating a patient with known lymphoma or pelvic malignancy.

The results of several investigations comparing CT and lymphography are similar (35-39). Each procedure has it advantages and limitations. Lymphography can demonstrate architectural changes in unenlarged nodes that appear normal on CT scans. Lymphographic patterns may suggest the etiology of lymphadenopathy, whereas CT demonstrates only nodal enlargement. CT, on the other hand, often shows the extent of lymphadenopathy to be considerably greater than is apparent on lymphography. CT displays upper abdominal and mesentheric modes that are not ordinarily opacified by lymphography (Figure 6).

Also, the condition of other organs of interest, such as spleen and liver, can be evaluated on CT scans. Furthermore, CT is easily and quickly accomplished while lymphography can be technically difficult, time consuming, and sometimes medically contraindicated. An approach to staging lymphoma that is evolving in some centers is to use CT as the initial modality. If lymphadenopathy is obvious on CT, the lymphogram can usually be avoided, but if the CT findings are negative or equivocal, a lymphogram is frequently required.

Other Abdominal Tumors

A variety of malignant neoplasms, mostly sarcomas, arise from the extra-organ tissues of the abdominal cavity. Many of these tumors occur in the retroperitoneal space where they may remain clinically obscure until they attain enormous size. Although conventional radiologic examinations are often of little value in detecting these tumors, CT provides accurate information regarding their presence, extent, composition and effect on adjacent structures (40,41).

112

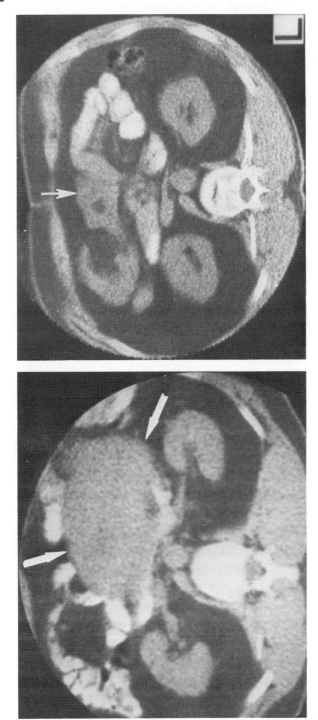

Figure 6 - A, B: Mesenteric lymphoma. A. A large mid-abdominal mass (arrows) of homogenous soft tissue density representing lymphocytic lymphoma confined to the nodes of the small bowel mesentery. B. Scan of the same region, four months later, after a course of radiation therapy shows marked diminution in size of the mass (arrows).

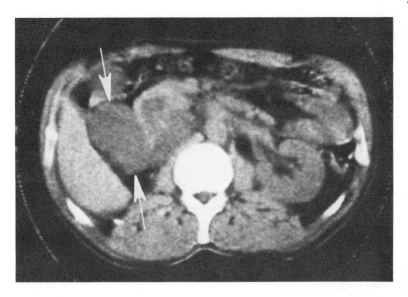

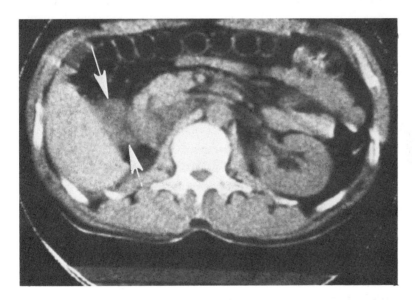

Figure 7 - A,B: Retroperitoneal liposarcoma. A. Scan seven months after resection of right retroperitoneal myxoid liposarcoma and involved right kidney shows a large recurrent tumor (arrows) in the right retroperitoneal space. B. Scan six months later, after course of chemotherapy, shows significant reduction in size of the lesion (arrows).

(Figure 7A from Stephens, DH, PF Sheedy, II, RR Hattery, B Williamson, Jr. Amer J Roentgenol 129:395, 1977 with permission)

For patients who receive irradiation or chemotherapy, CT is an excellent method to monitor the response of these neoplasms (Figure 7).

CT is likewise a method of choice to detect metastases and postoperative recurrences of tumors in locations, such as the mesentery, omentum, or abdominal wall, that are not visible on conventional radiographs (41-43). We have found CT to be especially useful to detect pelvic recurrences of rectosigmoid carcinoma following abdominoperineal resection (44).

SUMMARY

The role of CT relative to other imaging methods in the diagnosis of abdominal neoplasms is still under investigation. The relationships of CT to hepatic scintigraphy and to lymphography have been mentioned and are thoroughly discussed in other reports (16-18, 20, 35-39, 45, 46).

The relative efficacy of CT and ultrasonography is of particular interest and is somewhat more difficult to assess. Rapid technological advancements in both methods have tended to render comparative studies obsolete. Furthermore, results obtained at one institution are not necessarily applicable to another, as there are significant variations in methodology, experience, interpreter interest and patient population among different clinical settings. In our practice, CT has more consistently provided accurate information in the detection, evaluation and exclusion of most abdominal neoplasms, but neither method has been clearly superior to the other in all situations. Each method has its own advantages and disadvantages, and a variety of practical considerations may make one or the other the initial method of choice. Because CT and ultrasonography derive their images from different properties of tissues, their information is often complementary rather than competitive, and the results of both methods may be needed (18,26,46,47). Since the most appropriate choice of diagnostic procedures varies according to individual clinical circumstances, the patient's interests are often best served by preliminary consultation between the clinician and the radiologist.

REFERENCES

1. Schellinger, E, G DiChiro, SP Axelbaum, HL Twigg, RS Ledley, Early clinical experience with the ACTA scanner. Radiology 114:257, 1975

2. Alfidi, RJ, J Haaga, TF Meaney, WJ MacIntyre, L Gongales, R Tara, MG Zelch, M Boller, SA Cook, G Jelden, Computed tomography of the thorax and abdomen: a preliminary report. Radiology 117:257, 1975

3. Sagel, SS, RJ Stanley, RG Evens, Early experiences with motionless whole body computed tomography. Radiology 119:321, 1976

4. Stephens, DH, RR Hattery, Sheedy PF II, Computed tomography of the abdomen: early experience with the EMI body scanner. Radiology 119:331, 1976

5. Sheedy, PF, II, DH Stephens, RR Hattery, JR Muhm, GW Hartman, Computed tomography of the body: initial clinical trial with the EMI prototype. Amer J Roentgenol 127:23, 1976

6. Stanley, RJ, SS Sagel, RG Levitt, Computed tomography of the body: early trends in application and accuracy of the method. Amer J Roentgenol 127:53, 1976

7. Wittenberg, J, JT Ferrucci, Jr, Computed body tomography. Gastroenterology 74:287, 1978

8. Sheedy, PF, II, DH Stephens, RR Hattery, LR Brown, RL MacCarty, Computed tomography of abdominal organs. In: Advances in Internal Medicine, Vol 24, Stollerman, GH (ed), New York, Year Book Medical Publishers, 1979, p 455-479

9. Haaga, JR, RJ Alfidi, Precise biopsy localization by computed tomography. Radiology 118:603, 1976

10. Ferrucci, JT, Jr., J Wittenberg, CT biopsy of abdominal tumors: aids for lesion localization. Radiology 129:739, 1978

11. Jelden, GL, ES Chernak, A Rodriquez-Antunez, JR Haaga, PS Lavik, RS Dhaliwal, Further progress in CT scanning and computerized radiation therapy treatment planning. Amer J Roentgenol 127:179, 1976

12. Stewart, JR, LD Simpson, Computed tomography and the quality of radiation therapy. Amer J Roentgenol 129:943, 1977

13. Stephens, DH, PF Sheedy II, RR Hattery, RL MacCarty, Computed tomography of the liver. Amer J Roentgenol 128:579, 1977

14. Levitt, RG, SS Sagel, RJ Stanley, RG Jost, Accuracy of computed tomography of the liver and biliary tract. Radiology 124:123, 1977

15. Scherer, U, R Rainer, J Eisenburg, FW Schildberg, P Meister, J Lissner, Diagnostic accuracy of CT in circumscript liver disease. Amer J Roentgenol 130:711, 1978

16. Petasnick, JP, P Ram, DA Turner, EW Fordham, The relationship of computed tomography, gray-scale ultrasonography, and radionuclide imaging in the evaluation of hepatic masses. Seminars Nucl Med 9:8, 1979

17. MacCarty, RL, DH Stephens, RR Hattery, PF Sheedy, II, Hepatic imaging by computed tomography: a comparison with 99mTc - sulfur colloid, ultrasonography, and angiography. Radiol Clin N Amer 17:137, 1979

18. Snow, JH, Jr, HM Goldstein, S Wallace, Comparison of scintigraphy, sonography, and computed tomography in the evaluation of hepatic neoplasms. Amer J Roentgenol 132:915, 1979

19. Itai, Y, J Nishidawa, A Tasaka, Computed tomography in the evaluation of hepatocellular carcinoma. Radiology 131:165, 1979

20. Goldberg, HI, RA Filly, M Korobkin, AA Moss, HY Kressel, PW Callen, Capability of CT body scanning and ultrasonography to demonstrate the status of the biliary ductal system in patients with jaundice. Radiology 129:731, 1978

21. Haaga, JR, RJ Alfidi, TR Havrilla, R Tubbs, L Gonggales, TF Meaney, MA Corsi, Definitive role of CT scanning of the pancreas. Radiology 124:723, 1977

22. Stanley, RJ, SS Sagel, RG Levitt, Computed tomographic evaluation of the pancreas. Radiology 124:715, 1977

23. Sheedy, PF, II, DH Stephens, RR Hattery, RL MacCarty, Computed tomography in the evaluation of patients with suspected carcinoma of the pancreas: the second year's experience. Radiology 124:723, 1977

24. Sheedy, PF, II, DH Stephens, RR Hattery, RL MacCarty, B Williamson, Computed tomography of the pancreas. Radiol Clin N Amer 15:349, 1977

25. Moss, AA, HY Kressel, Computed tomography of the pancreas. Digestive Dis 22:1018, 1977

26. Lee, JKT, RJ Stanley, GL Melson, SS Sagel, Pancreatic imaging by ultrasound and computed tomography. Radiol Clin N Amer 17:105, 1979

27. Montagne, JP, HY Kressel, M Korobkin, AA Moss, Computed tomography of the normal adrenal glands. Amer J Roentgenol 130:963, 1978

28. Karstaldt, N, SS Sagel, RJ Stanley, GL Melson, RG Levitt, Computed tomography of the adrenal gland. Radiology 129:723, 1978

29. Dunnick, NR, EG Schaner, JL Doppman, CA Strott, JR Gill, N Javadpour, Computed tomography in adrenal tumors. Amer J Roentgenol 132:43, 1979

30. Reynes, CJ, R Churchill, R Moncada, L Love, Computed tomography of adrenal glands. Radiol Clin N Amer 17:91, 1979

31. Hattery, RR, B Williamson, DH Stephens, PF Sheedy, II, GW Hartman, Computed tomography of renal abnormalities. Radiol Clin N Amer 15:401, 1977

32. Sagel, SS, RJ Stanley, RG Levitt, G Geisse, Computed tomography of the kidneys. Radiology 124:359, 1977

33. Williamson, B, RR Hattery, DH Stephens, PF Sheedy, II, Computed tomography of the kidneys. Seminars Roentgenol 8:249, 1978

34. Love, L, CJ Reynes, R Churchill, R Moncade, Third generation CT scanning in renal disease. Radiol Clin N Amer 17:77, 1979

35. Schaner, EG, GL Head, JL Doppman, RC Young, Computed tomography in the diagnosis, staging and management of abdominal lymphoma. J Comput Assist Tomogr 1:176, 1977

36. Stephens, DH, B Williamson, PF Sheedy, II, RR Hattery, WE Miller, Computed tomography of the retroperitoneal space. Radiol Clin N Amer 15:377, 1977

37. Lee, JKT, RJ Stanley, SS Sagel, RG Levitt, Accuracy of computed tomography in detecting intra-abdominal and pelvic adenopathy in lymphoma. Amer J Roentgenol 131:311, 1978

38. Lee, JKT, RJ Stanley, SS Sagel, BL McClennan, Accuracy of CT in detecting intra-abdominal and pelvic lymph node metastases from pelvic cancers. Amer J Roentgenol 131:675, 1978

39. Zelch, MG, JR Haaga, Clinical comparison of computed tomography and lymphangiography for detection of retroperitoneal lymphadenopathy. Radiol Clin N Amer 17:157, 1979

40. Stephens, DH, PF Sheedy, II, RR Hattery, B Williamson, Diagnosis and evaluation of retroperitoneal tumors by computed tomography. Amer J Roentgenol 129:395, 1977

41. Carter, BL, RJ Wechsler, Computed tomography of the retroperitoneum and abdominal wall. Seminars in Roentgenol 13:201, 1978

42. Levitt, RG, SS Sagel, RJ Stanley, Detection of neoplastic involvement of the mesentery and omentum by computed tomography. Amer J Roentgenol 131:835, 1978

43. Bernardino, ME, BS Jing, S Wallace, Computed tomography diagnosis of mesenteric masses. Amer J Roentgenol 132:33, 1979

44. Williamson, B, Jr, RR Hattery, DH Stephens, PF Sheedy, II, Computed tomography of the pelvis following abdominoperineal resection for carcinoma of the rectum (in press)

45. MacCarty, RL, HW Wahner, DH Stephens, PF Sheedy, II, RR Hattery, Retrospective comparison of radionuclide scans and computed tomography of the liver and pancreas. Amer J Roentgenol 129:23, 1977

46. Bryan, PF, WW Dinn, Isodense masses on CT: differentiation by gray scale ultrasonography. Amer J Roentgenol 129:489, 1977

47. Levitt, RG, G Geisse, SS Sagel, RJ Stanley, RG Evens, RE Koehler, RG Jost, Complementary use of ultrasound and computed tomography in studies of the pancreas and kidney. Radiology 126:149, 1978

MANAGEMENT OF GASTRIC AND PANCREATIC CANCER

J.J. Gullo, M. Citron, F.P. Smith,
J.S. Macdonald and P.S. Schein
Vincent T. Lombardi Cancer Research Center
Washington, D.C.

GASTRIC CARCINOMA

Introduction

Cancer of the stomach has been declining in incidence over the past forty years. Nonetheless, it currently represents the sixth most common cause of cancer mortality in this country, accounting for 14,000 deaths per year. Greater than 23,000 cases can still be expected to be diagnosed annually (1). Surgical resection is the primary treatment for gastric cancer and currently is the only potentially curative therapy for this malignancy. In carcinomas of the antrum or body of the stomach, subtotal gastrectomy is the usual operative procedure; whereas, in primary lesions of the cardia, a total gastrectomy and distal esophagectomy should be performed. The operative mortality is approximately 10% for the subtotal procedure and may be as high as 20% for the total gastrectomy (2).

Prognostic Determinants

Pathological examination of the surgical specimen is of prognostic value. In those instances in which there is a small distal lesion with no evidence of vascular, lymphatic or serosal involvement, patients have approximately a 50% chance for five year disease free survival. When regional lymph nodes are involved, the probability of five year survival after surgical resection alone drops to approximately 15% (2). Linitis plastica also carries a poor prognosis with less than 10% of patients surviving more than five years. In the United States, the vast majority of patients with gastric cancer are detected with advanced stages of disease with an overall five year survival of 7-12% (2). Therefore, many of these individuals will be candidates for non-surgical modalities of management. Patients with surgically incurable gastric cancer present two clinical pictures: (1) unresectable regional progression, or (2) hematogenous metastases to the liver, lung or bone. Patients with locally advanced disease may be candidates for regional forms of therapy, such as radiation with or without chemotherapy, whereas the patients with advanced systemic disease will require systemic chemotherapy.

Therapy for Locally Advanced Disease

Radiation Therapy. Radiation therapy alone, in patients with locally unresectable or recurrent gastric cancer, may be useful for palliation of pain and obstruction but has not prolonged survival. Investigators at the Mayo Clinic (2), however, have demonstrated that radiation therapy combined with 5-fluorouracil can afford these patients a modest (statistically significant) improvement in survival. Patients received 3750 rads of split course radiation therapy with either 5-fluorouracil for the first 3 days of each course or intravenous placebo. Patients treated with the combination of 5-FU and 3750 rads lived for an average of 14 months, compared to 5.9 months for patients treated with 3750 rads alone (p=0.05).

Chemotherapy. Recent data suggests that chemotherapy may be at least as effective as radiation therapy in the management of patients found to have locally recurrent or unresectable disease. The Gastrointestinal Tumor Study Group (3) compared chemotherapy with 5-FU and methyl-CCNU to a combined modality approach in which 500 rads of regional radiation was given in two split courses with 500 mg/m^2 5-FU administered IV on the first 3 days of each radiation course and then followed by 5-FU and methyl-CCNU. Ninety-six patients were stratified by histology, location of primary tumor, surgical resectability and extent of residual tumor prior to randomization. The median time to disease progression for the group receiving irradiation followed by chemotherapy was 18 weeks while it was 23 weeks for the group receiving chemotherapy alone. The median survival differences were significant; 40 weeks for radiation and chemotherapy compared to 71 weeks for the chemotherapy group (p=0.005). Furthermore, the radiation therapy group experienced greater treatment related toxicity; 64% compared to 40% (p=0.05) experienced a greater reduction in performance status (p=0.06) and had more progressive weight loss (p=0.05). This study suggests that the major emphasis in treating patients with locally advanced gastric cancer should now be placed on the use of effective combination chemotherapy. Therefore, in this subgroup of patients, combination chemotherapy should now be considered the standard to which innovative forms of radiation therapy such as high Linear Energy Transfer (LET) therapy and intra-operative irradiation should be compared.

Chemotherapy of Disseminated Disease

General. Many patients with adenocarcinoma of the stomach present with disseminated disease or develop metastases which make them candidates for systemic cytotoxic chemotherapy. Table 1 reviews the reported activity of single agents in gastric cancer. Only those drugs which have undergone Phase II trial in greater than fifteen patients are included.

Table 1. Single agent activity in gastric cancer
(>15 patients on study)

Drug	% Response	Reference
5-Fluorouracil	21	4
Mitomycin-C	20	6
BCNU	18	10
Methyl-CCNU	8	11
Adriamycin	30	5
Hydroxyurea	19	13
DTIC	13	14
Mechlorethane	13	15
Chlorambucil	17	16

5-Fluorouracil. The most completely evaluated drug is the fluorinated pyrimidine, 5-fluorouracil, which has been tested in over four hundred patients (4,5). The most common reported schedule is the loading course method in which the drug is administered intravenously for four days followed by half-doses every other day until toxicity is produced. This is followed by weekly maintenance therapy or repeated loading courses at monthly intervals. The overall response rate for patients treated with loading dose 5-FU is 21% (4). A small number of patients have received weekly intravenous treatment with a similar response. The median durations of 5-FU response have ranged from three to six months.

Mitomycin-C. The secondmost actively investigated drug in advanced gastric cancer has been mitomycin-C (5,6). This antibiotic was first developed in Japan where clinical trials suggested an overall objective response rate of 35% (7). The initial experience in the United States showed that Mitomycin-C, administered on a daily schedule, produced significant and delayed myelosuppression with cumulative and persistent injury to the bone marrow (8). Inadvertent extravasation resulted in a severe inflammatory reaction. Drug-related deaths occurred in 11% of the patients, and the initial study (8) in this country documented an objective response rate of only 18%. More recent experience has shown an overall response rate for mitomycin-C in gastric cancer of 15-30% (6). There has been renewed enthusiasm for this drug, particularly with the demonstration that treatment at six to eight week intervals results in manageable hematological toxicity while retaining therapeutic activity (9).

Nitrosoureas. The chloroethyl-nitrosourea, BCNU, has been actively investigated for efficacy against advanced gastric cancer (5). Objective remissions were observed in six of 33 patients treated for a response rate of 18% with a four month duration of response (10). The methyl-nitrosourea, MeCCNU, has also been tested and found to have a response rate of 8% (11).

Anthracyclines. The anthracycline antibiotic, adriamycin, a drug with a wide spectrum of antitumor activity, was found to produce a response rate of 30% in gastric cancer (5). A recent study by the Gastrointestinal Tumor Study Group (GITSG) obtained a somewhat lower but appreciable response of 25%. This drug has been of considerable interest because of its potential use in combination chemotherapy and data suggesting that adriamycin may have second line activity. The Eastern Cooperative Oncology Group demonstrated that 19% of patients who had previously been treated with either 5-FU + mitomycin-C or 5-FU + methyl-CCNU responded to adriamycin (12). Adriamycin can thus be used as "salvage" treatment for patients failing primary chemotherapy.

Other Agents. Other single agents including hydroxyurea, DTIC and a limited number of alkylating agents (13-16) have been reported to have activity of less than 20% in advanced gastric cancer cases but may be worthy of further investigation. In general, all single agents used in gastric cancer shared the disadvantage of low response rates and short duration of response (3-5 months). For these reasons, single agent chemotherapy tends to be of limited benefit to the patient. Therefore, polychemotherapy in patients with stomach cancer is being viewed with increasing interest.

Combination Chemotherapy. Table 2 reviews the combination chemo-therapeutic regimens that have been tested in 10 or more patients. As can be seen, the drug combinations use the limited number of individually active agents.

Table 2. Combination chemotherapy of gastric cancer
($\geq$ 10 patients on study)

Drug Regimen	% Response	Reference
5-FU + adriamycin + mitomycin-C	50	22
	38	23
	33	18
5-FU + BCNU	41	
5-FU + adriamycin	35	
5-FU + mitomycin	34	
5-FU + methyl-CCNU	40	11
	10	21
	24	12
	21	17
5-FU + cytosine arabinoside, mitomycin-C	55	19
	38	20
	21	21
5-FU + adriamycin + methyl-CCNU	30	18
5-FU - ICRF - 159 + methyl-CCNU	23	18

The most extensively evaluated regimens in the United States have used 5-FU in combination with either BCNU or methyl-CCNU (10,11).

BCNU + 5-FU. The combination of 5-FU and BCNU was compared to each drug used as a single agent (10). All drugs were given intravenously as follows: 5-FU alone, 13.5 mg/kg/day for five days; BCNU alone, 50 mg/m^2/day for five days; and 5-FU + BCNU, 10 mg/kg/day and 40 mg/m^2/day for five days respectively. Objective responses to therapy were 29% for 5-FU alone, 17% for BCNU alone, and 41% for 5-FU + BCNU. Long term survival for the combination was superior to 5-FU alone and median survival for the combination and 5-FU alone was significantly better than BCNU alone.

Methyl-CCNU + 5-FU. The Eastern Cooperative Oncology Group has conducted a controlled randomized trial in advanced gastric cancer comparing the combination of 5-FU and methyl-CCNU with methyl-CCNU used alone. The combination consisted of 5-FU at 300 mg/m^2/day intravenously with methyl-CCNU at 175 mg/m^2 given orally on the first day; this regimen was repeated at seven week intervals. Methyl-CCNU alone was 200 mg/m^2 given in a single oral dose and repeated at seven week intervals. The combination produced a 40% response rate and was definitely superior to methyl-CCNU alone, which produced 8% response (p=0.05) (11). There was significant survival benefit reported for the patients treated with the combination. These studies demonstrate an improvement in survival for patients with gastric cancer through the use of chemotherapy.

There is a suggestion that the 40% response rate for 5-FU + methyl-CCNU may not be entirely reproducible. Baker et al (17) for the Southwest Oncology Group reported a comparison of 5-FU and 5-FU + methyl-CCNU and noted that the objective response rate in 29 patients with gastric cancer for the combination was only 20.7%. This was not different from the response rate produced by 5-FU alone. However, the latter study used 5-FU in a relatively low dose of 400 mg/m^2 IV weekly rather than the IV loading dose as in the previous studies. Recent results, from a GITSG comparative study of a loading dose of 5-FU and methyl-CCNU (FuMe) reveals that the combination of 5-FU and methyl-CCNU produces a response of 10%, whereas the combinations of 5-FU, adriamycin + mitomycin-C (FAM) or 5-FU, adriamycin + methyl-CCNU (FAMe) have a response rate of 33% and 30% respectively. The median survival for FuMe was 23 weeks as compared to that of 29 weeks for FAM and 39 weeks for FAMe (18).

5-FU, Mitomycin-C and Cytosine Arabinoside. Based upon evidence of synergism in rodent tumor, the combination of 5-FU, mitomycin-C + cytosine arabinoside underwent clinical trial in Japan where a 55% response rate was reported for 27 patients (19). However, in attempts to confirm these data, a more modest remission rate of 38% was seen in one study (20) and 21% in another (21).

5-FU, Adriamycin and Mitomycin-C (FAM). An evaluation of the combination of flurouracil, adriamycin and mitomycin-C (FAM) revealed an overall response rate of 50% in 36 patients with advanced gastric cancer (22). Responses were seen in both metastatic liver disease and large abdominal masses, and response of responders was 13 months compared with three months for non-responders (figure 1).

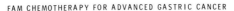

FAM CHEMOTHERAPY FOR ADVANCED GASTRIC CANCER

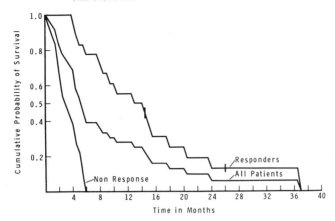

Figure 1: Survival curves comparing responding and non-responding patients

FAM was well tolerated with the major toxicities being moderate myelosuppression (WBC <1.5 x 10^3/mm^3 in 17% of patients and platelet count <50 x 10^3/mm^3 in 31% of patients). There were no drug related deaths or serious morbidity.

In an updated series of 61 patients (including the above) treated at the Vincent T. Lombardi Cancer Research Center in collaboration with Professor Lagarde in Bordeaux and Professor Barron in Paris, 38% achieved a partial response (23). The median survival has not yet been attained. The FAM regimen is currently undergoing Phase III trials in the GITSG to define whether this treatment program is capable of improving survival when compared to other combination chemotherapy regimens (23). The initial results show a 38% remission rate with a median survival for FAM treated patients of at least 34 weeks. This median survival is currently superior to 19 week median survival produced by the other regimen in this study, 5-FU + ICRF-159 + methyl-CCNU (18).

In earlier trials, 5-FU + adriamycin (24) and 5-FU + mitomycin (12) were demonstrated to produce response rates of 35% and 34% respectively. Prospective comparisons of FAM to these regimens are therefore warranted to determine if the full FAM combination is necessary. Phase III studies of FAM in advanced gastric cancer have also been initiated by Cancer and Acute Leukemia Group B, the Southwest Oncology Group and the Eastern Cooperative Oncology

Group. The results of these group studies will establish the magnitude of activity for this combination. At this time the data indicate that FAM is an active and well tolerated regimen for the treatment of stomach cancer.

Future Directions for Gastric Cancer

The documented activity of combination chemotherapy allows two approaches for the treatment of gastric cancer. First, it is reasonable to test regimens such as FAM in the therapy of early stages of the disease. Prospectively controlled surgical adjuvant studies are certainly appropriate. Aggressive combination chemotherapy could also be applied to patients with locally unresectable disease. The second approach to be taken in patients with advanced gastric cancer is to modify the active combinations by either substitution of agents that produce less toxicities or by the addition of agents having the potential for pharmacologic synergism with established regimens. Hopefully, such new combinations would produce more responses and could be applied to improve long term survival from gastric cancer.

CANCER OF THE PANCREAS

Introduction

Cancer of the pancreas is the second most common gastrointestinal malignancy and the fourth leading cause of cancer deaths in the United States (25,26). In spite of advances in diagnostic and surgical techniques, overall survival for patients with this disease remains dismally low. Surgical resection is still the only therapy with potential for cure; however, the operative mortality of resection in recent series exceeds the five year survival rate of less than 4% (27). More aggressive surgical procedures have only resulted in prohibitive morbidity (28).

Although many patients will have localized disease at the time of laparotomy, less than 10 - 15% of such cases will be resectable due to frequent involvement of regional nodes, as well as important vascular or neural structures (29,30). Therefore, the vast majority of patients will require some form of effective postoperative therapy. In locally advanced, non-resectable pancreatic carcinoma, radiotherapy or combined modality therapy has been the standard form of management. With metastatic disease that cannot be encompassed by a reasonable radiation port, systemic chemotherapy will be required. In this report, we will review and update the available information for management of "surgically incurable" carcinoma of the pancreas.

Locally Advanced Carcinoma Of The Pancreas

Interstitial Irradiation. Probably the first treatment of a patient with pancreatic cancer was by Upcott, who in 1892 reported placing 5 mg of radium into a cholecystostomy after surgical removal of a carcinoma of the Ampulla of Vater (31). Thirteen years later, the next patient treated in this manner survived for twenty months (32). Handley began true interstitial implantation in 1925 (33). Seven patients were treated with doses ranging from 675-1800 mg - hours. Four died within twenty-five days of surgery; one patient reported palliation of pain. Although a few long term survivors were reported, no histologic confirmation of malignancy was available in these cases. Pack and McNeer reported the first permanent implantation of gold-filtered radon seeds into three patients with pancreatic cancer in 1938 (34). Fortner et al (35) in a retrospective analysis suggested that interstitial implantation of [121] or [192] IR appeared as effective as external beam in increasing median survival and relieving jaundice. Eighty percent of patients treated with interstitial irradiation to a tumor dose of 16,000 R obtained relief of pain compared to 62% of those receiving external beam therapy. The use of interstitial irradiation is currently under further investigation at the Thomas Jefferson University, Massachusetts General Hospital and other centers. If these studies prove promising, a prospectively randomized Phase III study comparing interstitial to external beam radiotherapy should be encouraged.

External Beam Irradiation. Richards was the first to report on the use of external beam irradiation for pancreatic cancers (36). Two patients with biopsy-proven, locally unresectable disease were treated, both experiencing relief of pain and weight gain. At the time of his report, both patients were clinically free of disease with good performance status at 10 and 27 months. Moertel and Childs reported a retrospective analysis of 62 patients with locally unresectable pancreatic carcinoma treated conventionally to a dose of 3,500 rads (27,38). They concluded that survival in these patients was not significantly different from those of the matched untreated "controls." Billingsly et al (39) arrived at similar conclusions in a retrospective analysis of 13 patients treated with cobalt therapy in doses ranging from 700-4,000 rads.

Haslam et al (40) treated 29 patients to doses as high as 6,700 rads in 10 weeks in a double split course fashion using [60] Co teletherapy. Many of the patients ahcieving survival benefit had concurrent chemotherapy. The median survival of the patients treated with radiation alone was 8 months, while for the group receiving radiation and chemotherapy, the median survival was 11 months.

Fifty percent of the patients received good palliative results but morbidity approached 30%, especially with the combined technique. Dobelbower et al suggested that even higher doses of radiation, 6,000-7,000 rads, were necessary to gain control for unresectable primary (41). Survival in Dobelbower's patients appeared better than those reported by Haslam. However, as in the latter study, many of the patients also received chemotherapy which appeared to confer an improved survival (12 vs. 15 months).

Chemotherapy and Radiation Therapy. Chemotherapy, when combined with radiation therapy, has a proven role in the treatment of the locally advanced stage of pancreatic cancer. Moertel and co-workers had reported that the addition of 5-fluorouracil (5-FU) to 3,500-4,000 rads of split course regional radiation could result in improved patient survival (42,43). 5-fluorouracil was administered intravenously in daily doses of 15 mg/kg on the first 3 days of the course of radiation. This was prospectively compared to the same dose of radiation plus placebo. Sixty-four patients participated in the study, which demonstrated a statistically improved mean survival in the 5-FU treated group; 10.4 months versus 6.3 months (p=0.05).

In 1974, the GITSG initiated a controlled trial comparing 6000 rads photon irradiation with 6,000 rads and 5-FU and 4,000 rads and 5-FU for patients with locally advanced pancreatic cancer (44). The maximum allowable radiation port was 20 cm x 20 cm. The radiation therapy was delivered in split courses of 2,000 rads in two weeks each separated by a two week rest and recovery interval (figure 2).

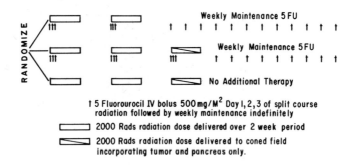

Figure 2: Treatment schema for GITSG study comparing radiotherapy alone with radiotherapy plus 5-FU for unresectable carcinoma of the pancreas.

5-Fluorouracil was administered intravenously at a dose of 500 mg/m^2 on the first three days of each course of radiation, and continued weekly thereafter until progression in patients receiving the combined modality. It soon became apparent that the regimen of 6,000 rads of irradiation was producing a significantly inferior survival when compared to each of the combined modality forms of treatment (46). The median time to progression with high dose irradiation alone was 13 weeks compared to 28 weeks with 4,000 rads plus 5-FU and 32 weeks with 6,000 rads plus 5-FU. The survivals at that time point in the study demonstrated an 18 week median for 6,000 rads alone compared to 35 weeks with the two combined approaches (figure 3).

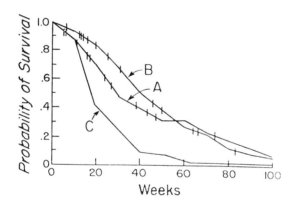

Figure 3: Survival curve for patients receiving either 4000R radiotherapy plus 5-FU (A) or 6000R radiotherapy plus 5-FU (B) or radiotherapy alone (C).

The high dose radiation therapy arm was terminated, but the study was continued for evaluation of the two doses of irradiation combined with 5-FU until May, 1978. At the same time multivariate analysis of prognostic determinants of survival were undertaken. An initial poor performance status (ECOG 2-3), vomiting as a pretreatment symptom, and a tumor with a scirrhous reaction were found to be significant negative variables. The corrected median survival for 4,000 rads plus 5-FU is 31 weeks, compared to 39 weeks with 6,000 rads and 5-FU; the difference is close to statistical significance (44).

It must be acknowledged that this form of therapy, while producing an improved survival, is not curative. The projected survival at two years is 10% or less. This study has conclusively demonstrated the importance of 5-FU as an adjuvant to irradiation. The principal role of this drug in the combined modality regimen is not fully understood; it may function as radiation sensitizer as well as a direct acting cytotoxic agent. Nonetheless, 5-FU with 4,000 or 6,000 rads should be considered standard therapy for locally advanced pancreatic cancer to which newer forms of management must eventually be compared.

Other Radiation Therapy Approaches. The combination of 5-FU and fast neutron therapy has been studied at the Vincent T. Lombardi Cancer Research Center in cooperation with the Mid-Atlantic Neutron Therapy Association. Fast neutrons have a theoretical advantage over conventional photon therapy in that they do not require oxygen for effectiveness and thus may be more appropriate therapy for large, deepseated tumor masses with anoxic centers (46). Seventeen patients with locally advanced pancreatic carcinoma have been treated with 1,716 rads of 15 MEV fast neutrons with or without 5-FU at 375 mg/m^2 to 500 mg/m^2 administered daily on the first and last three days of radiation therapy (47). Thirteen patients had followable disease, and partial responses were recorded in 6 (46%) with median duration of survival of 13 months (range 6 - 22+) in responders. The median survival for non-responders was 4 months (range 2-5+). Of particular note is that 2 of the responders are alive at 22 months and 18 months and the latter patient on re-exploration for gastrointestinal bleeding was found to have no surgical evidence of residual tumor (unpublished data).

Intraoperative radiation therapy and pi-meson therapy are currently underway at Howard University and the Northern California Oncology Group respectively (48). These and other innovative attempts at combined modality therapy are clearly to be encouraged. Newer radiosensitizers such as misonidazole with conventional external beam and other forms of irradiation should be investigated and compared with the combination of 5-FU and therapeutic radiation to test the role of cytotoxic effect of 5-FU in combined modality.

Therapy of Advanced Pancreatic Cancer

General. Relatively few anticancer agents have undergone adequate testing for patients with advanced pancreatic cancer (49-52). Furthermore, Phase II studies designed to test the activity of new drugs require that the population studied has measurable disease. This, to date, has not been the case in patients with pancreatic carcinoma. The advent of pancreatic sonography and computed tomography may, however, in part, correct this deficiency. In addition, the disease frequently leads to rapid debilitation, often accompanied by severe pain, anorexia, weight loss and malabsorption (51,53). This problem further contributes to the lack of suitable patients for adequate clinical trials.

Therefore, the majority of patients that fulfill the necessary criteria usually have massive tumor burden and an extremely poor performance status accompanied by pain, hepatic dysfunction and cachexia. These patients cannot tolerate a toxic regimen; they are the worst class of patients in whom to assess therapeutic effectiveness of a new treatment.

Single Agent Chemotherapy in Pancreatic Cancer. 5-fluorouracil has been the most extensively studied drug for advanced pancreatic cancer (52). Response rates have varied between 0 and 67% (54). Carter et al (50) reported a response rate of 28% in a collective series of 212 patients. More current trials have reported response rates of approximately 20% (52,53).

Mitomycin-C, a drug first introduced in Japan, has an activity of approximately 27% in a collective series of patients (50). This drug fell into disfavor in this country due to severe problems of marrow hypoplasia (56). However, with more attention to scheduling and dose of the drug, it can be administered safely as a single agent as well as in combination with other drugs.

The chloroethylnitrosoureas have been tested extensively in pancreatic cancer at the Mayo Clinic (57) and by the Eastern Cooperative Oncology Group (58) and have shown a meager 9-13% activity as single agents. Streptozotocin, a naturally occurring methylnitrosourea is a potent toxin for pancreatic islet Beta cells in animals. This property has been exploited clinically in the treatment of islet cell carcinoma (59). Activity in adenocarcinoma of the pancreas as a single agent is unclear but in small trials it has had objective response rates of 30-50% (60,61).

The GITSG has tested several agents for single agent activity (62,63). Adriamycin was found to have a 13% activity in previously untreated patients. Other agents tested by them and found to have essentially no activity in this disease include methotrexate, actinomycin-D, ICRF-159, galactitol, a B-dioxythioguanosine.

Yunis et al (64) tested the sensitivity of two cell lines of pancreatic cancer (MiA Pa Ca-Z and PANC-1) to L-asparaginase. They found that L-asparaginase produced significant growth inhibition which appeared to be specific since there was no effect on human breast cancer and melanoma cell lines. A subsequent clinical trial at the University of Miami was disappointing, with no therapeutic activity demonstrated.

There is little information available in the use of alkylating agents, but a few small trials have suggested some activity for chlorambucil, Cytoxan, and mechlorethamine (65-67).

Combination Chemotherapy in Pancreatic Cancer. Kovach (10) and co-workers randomized 82 patients with advanced pancreatic carcinoma to receive either 5-FU alone at a dose of 13 mg/kg/day IV x 5 d every 5 weeks, or BCNU at 10 mg/kg/day x 5 days every 5 weeks. A third group of patients received a combination of 5-FU 10 mg/kg/day and BCNU at a dose of 40 mg/m^2/day x 5 days every 5 weeks. While BCNU exhibited no activity in the 21 patients treated and 5-FU had activity of only 16%, the combination surprisingly had a response rate of 33%. Despite this, there was no survival benefit to this regimen as compared to the single agent activity.

Waddell (68) employed 5-FU plus daily oral testolactone $\pm$ spironolactone in 13 patients with advanced pancreatic carcinoma. The median survival of this group was 21 months. Testolactone was employed because of in-vitro evidence suggesting it had an inhibiting effect on purine synthesis, thus accounting for the enhancement in the activity of 5-FU when the lactone was added. In a prospective randomized trial conducted by the ECOG, however, spironolactone added nothing to the therapeutic efficacy of 5-FU or 5-FU + streptozotocin (69).

Buroker (70), in a randomized trial employing 5-FU given as a loading dose by continuous infusion over 5 days in conjunction with either mitomycin-C or methyl-CCNU, found the regimen of 5-FU and mitomycin-C to have a response rate of pf 30% as compared to 17% for 5-FU and methyl-CCNU (p=0.03). In this study, 5-FU was given at a dose of 1000 mg/m^2/day x 5 days every 8 weeks, mitomycin 20 mg/m^2 every 8 weeks or methyl-CCNU 175/mg/m^2 every 8 weeks.

In 1974, the Vincent T. Lombardi Cancer Research Center initiated a Phase II trial of a combination of 3 drugs, which at the time of the study design had reported single agent activity in pancreatic cancer; streptozotocin, mitomycin-C and 5-FU (SMF) (71). SMF was administered in 8 week cycles, streptozotocin 1 gm/m^2 IV and 5-FU 600mg/m^2 on weeks 1,2, 5 and 6, mitomycin-C on week 1 only (table 3); the cycle was repeated on week 9.

Table 3. SMF for advanced pancreatic carcinoma

Drug and Dosage	Week No.								
	1	2	3	4	5	6	7	8	9
Streptozotocin									
1 gm/m^2 IV	X	X			X	X			X
Mitomycin-C									
10 mg/m^2 IV	X								X
5-Fluorouracil									
600 mg/m^2 IV	X	X			X	X			X

One of the important innovations incorporated into the regimen was the use of mitomycin-C by the intermittent schedule. Twenty-three consecutive cases with advanced measurable pancreatic cancer were entered into this program. Ten of 23 (43%) achieved an objective response with one patient demonstrating a complete response with regression of biopsy-proven hepatic metastases. The responders demonstrated a median survival of 10 months as compared to 3 months for the non-responders. This was statistically significant (p=0.01) (figure 4).

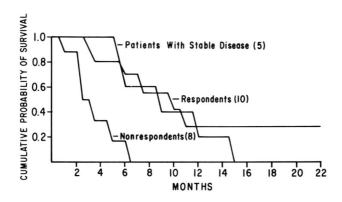

Figure 4: Survival curves for patients treated with SMF for pancreatic carcinoma.

The median survival of all cases was 6 months. Four of the 23 (17%) cases studied lived one year or longer. One patient who presented with biopsy-proven hepatic metastases and achieved a complete response documented by negative repeated liver biopsies is alive and free of clinical evidence of disease at 3.5 years from initiation of SMF therapy (unpublished data). It is important to recognize that the median performance status (PS) in this group of patients was 1, that is, symptomatic but ambulatory. Two patients had PS of 3 or were bedridden for greater than 50% of the time and only 1 patient was 100% bedridden. Thus, the majority of study cases were of good performance status; this stands in contrast to other treatment series in which debilitated patients have predominated.

Aberhalden et al (72) have obtained similar results to the SMF regimen with the combination of 5-FU (500 mg/m^2/day IV x 5), streptozotocin 300 mg/m^2/day IV x 5 with mitomycin-C 10 mg/m^2 IV administered every 8 weeks. An objective response was recorded in 5/16 (31%) of patients treated. The 2 drug combination of 5-FU and streptozotocin obtained a 21% response rate in their series. Thus, the combination of streptozotocin, mitomycin-C and 5-FU appears to have enhanced activity in pancreatic cancer and merits comparative study in Phase III trails in patients with locally unresectable disease. The nausea and vomiting produced by streptozotocin is a negative aspect of this program, however.

Following the demonstration that adriamycin had independent activity for advanced pancreatic cancer, the Vincent T. Lombardi Cancer Research Center initiated a pilot study of the FAM regimen of 5-FU, adriamycin and mitomycin-C (73). In this regimen (table 4), 5-FU is administered intravenously on weeks 1, 2, 5 and 6; adriamycin 30 mg/m^2 IV on weeks 1 and 5; and mitomycin-C 10 mg/m^2 IV on week 1.

Table 4.   The FAM regimen

Drug and Dosage	Week No.								
	1	2	3	4	5	6	7	8	9
5-Fluorouracil 600 mg/m^2 IV	X	X			X	X			X
Adriamycin 30 mg/m^2 IV	X				X				X
Mitomycin-C 10 mg/m^2 IV	X								X

This cycle is repeated on week 9. FAM had been previously tested in patients with advanced gastric cancer with a remission rate of 50% (22) and in a larger series of 38% (23). From January, 1977 through July, 1978, 37 patients with pancreatic cancer have been treated with this regimen. Twenty-five of these patients with advanced measurable disease are available for response evaluation. The median performance status in this group of patients was 2 with one-quarter of the patients having performance status 3. Ten of the 25 patients (40%) have obtained a partial response with a median survival in excess of 9 months for responders (p=.01) (73). The median survival for the entire group in this study is currently being evaluated. On initial evaluation, this regimen produces appreciably less gastrointestinal toxicity than the SMF combination. A Phase III evaluation of these two regimens is now in progress in the GITSG and is to be initiated by the CALGB.

Conclusion

Gastric cancer, although decreasing in incidence in this country, represents an important neoplasm ranking sixth in cancer mortality statistics. The majority of patients present with disease warranting systemic therapy. The GITSG study of locally advanced disease suggests that combination chemotherapy alone is superior to radiation with chemotherapy and must now be considered the standard for comparison in Phase III trials in this stage of gastric malignancy. New combinations such as FAM appear very promising and demonstrate this tumor to be both responsive and with apparent survival benefit resulting in responders. This encouraging data warrants the Phase III studies now in progress and consideration of the use of the combintion in the "adjuvant" setting.

Progress in pancreatic cancer has been less impressive in spite of this tumor's increasing importance. Its incidence has risen steadily over the past 3 to 4 decades and currently represents the fourth leading cause of cancer deaths in this country. In locally advanced disease, combined modality therapy with 5-FU and 4,000 or 6,000 rads is the accepted management, and appear to give the patient a small survival advantage. Newer forms of radiation such as particulate irradiation and intraoperative therapy are to be encouraged since the outlook for these patients remains bleak. There has not been adequate testing of single agents or combination chemotherapy in patients with advanced disease. Pilot and Phase II studies with SMF and FAM have appeared encouraging in our hands with response rates of approximately 40%. Phase III evaluation is needed. It is imperative to pursue innovative therapeutic courses in these patients to improve the dismal statistics currently generated for patients with carcinoma of the pancreas.

136

REFERENCES

1. Silverberg, E, Cancer statistics, 1977. Ca 27:26-41, 1977
2. Moertel, CG, Stomach cancer. In: Cancer Medicine, Holland, JF, E Frei III (eds), Philadelphia, Lea and Febiger, 1973, p 1527-1541
3. Schein, PS, D Childs, A controlled evaluation of combined modality therapy (5000 rad, 5-FU + MeCCNU) vs. 5-FU - MeCCNU alone for locally unresectable gastric cancer. Proc Amer Soc Clin Onc 19:329, 1978
4. Comis, RL, SK Carter, Integration of chemotherapy into combined modality treatment of solid tumors. III. Gastric cancer. Cancer Treat Rev 1:221-228, 1974
5. Moertel, CG, Chemotherapy of gastrointestinal cancer. Clin Gastroenterol 5:777-793, 1976
6. Moore, GF, IDJ Bross, R Ausman, Effects of mitomycin-C (NSC 26980) in 346 patients with advanced cancer. Cancer Chemother Rep 52:675-684, 1968
7. Frank, W, AE Osterberg, Mitomycin-C (NSC 26989. An evaluation of the Japanese reports. Cancer Chemother Rep 9:114-119, 1960
8. Jones, R, and Cooperating Investigators, Mitomycin-C - A preliminary report of studies of human pharmacology and initial therapeutic trial. Cancer Chemother Rep 2:3-7, 1959
9. Baker, L, EM Caoili, VK Izbick, et al, A comparative study of mitomycin-C and porfiromycin. Proc Amer Soc Clin Onc 15:182, 1974
10. Kovach, JS, CG Moertel, AJ Schutt, A controlled study of combined 1,3-bis(2-chloroethyl)-1-nitrosourea and 5-fluorouracil therapy for advanced gastric and pancreatic cancer. Cancer 33:563-567, 1974
11. Moertel, CG, JA Mettelman, RF Bakermeier, et al, Sequential and combination chemotherapy of advanced gastric cancer. Cancer 38:678-682, 1976
12. Eastern Cooperative Oncology Group, Personal communication, December, 1978
13. Livingston, RB, SK Carter, Single Agents in Cancer Chemotherapy. New York, IFI/Plenum, 1970
14. Goldsmith, MA, MA Friedman, SK Carter, Clinical brochure, 5-(3-3-dimethyl-1-triazeno) imidazole carboxamide (DTIC, DIC), National Cancer Institute, Bethesda, Maryland, 1972
15. Hurley, JD, EH Ellison, LL Carey, Treatment of advanced cancer of the gastrointestinal tract with antitumor agents. Gastroenterol 41:557-562, 1961

16. Moore, G, I Bross, R Ausman, et al, Effects of chlorambucil (NSC 3088) in 374 patients with advanced cancer. Cancer Chemother Rep 52:661-666, 1968

17. Baker, LH, RW Tolley, R Matter, et al, Phase III comparison of the treatment of advanced gastrointestinal cancer with bolus weekly 5-FU vs. methyl-CCNU plus bolus weekly 5-FU. Cancer 38:1-7, 1976

18. Gastrointestinal Tumor Study Group, Minutes of meeting, February, 1979, San Diego, California, p 55-60

19. Kazua, O, S Junita, M Nishimura, et al, Combination therapy with mitomycin-C (NSC 26980), 5-fluorouracil (NSC 19893) and cytosine arabinoside (NSC 63878) for advanced cancer in man. Cancer Chemother Rep 56:373-385, 1972

20. DeJager, GB, GB Magill, RB Golbey, et al, Mitomycin-C, 5-fluorouracil and cytosine arabinoside (MFC) in gastrointestinal cancer. Proc Amer Soc Clin Onc 15:178, 1974

21. Gastrointestinal Tumor Study Group, Minutes of meeting, February, 1978, Miami, Florida, p 43

22. Macdonald, JS, PV Woolley, T Smythe, et al, 5-fluorouracil, adriamycin, and mitomycin-C (FAM) combination chemotherapy in the treatment of advanced gastric cancer. Cancer 44:42-47, 1979

23. Macdonald, JS, PS Schein, PV Woolley, et al, 5-fluorouracil (5-FU), mitomycin-C (MMC), and Adriamycin (ADR) FAM combination chemotherapy results in 61 patients. Proc Amer Soc Clin Onc 20:396, 1979

24. Brugarolas, Personal communication, December, 1978

25. Holmes, FF, S Olson, C Lash, et al, Cancer data service: pancreatic carcinoma distantly metastatic at diagnosis, 1945-1974. J Kans Med Soc 78:472-473, 1977

26. Macdonald, JS, L Widerlite, PS Schein, Current diagnosis and management of pancreatic carcinoma. J Natl Cancer Inst 56:1093-1099, 1976

27. Borgelt, BB, RR Dobelbower, Jr, KA Strubler, Betatron therapy for unresectable pancreatic cancer. Amer J Surg 135:76-80, 1978

28. Drapanas, T, Regional resection for pancreatic carcinoma. Surgery 73:321-322, 1973

29. McDermott, MV, MK Bantlett, Pancreaticoduodenal cancer. New Engl J Med 248:927-931, 1953

30. Gudjonsson, B, EM Livstone, HM Spiro, Cancer of the pancreas: diagnostic accuracy and survival statistics. Cancer 42:2494-2506, 1978

138

31. Upcott, H, Tumors of the ampulla of vater. Amer Surg 56:710-725, 1912
32. Abell, I, Carcinoma of the papilla of vater. South Med J 17:24-27, 1924
33. Handley, WS, Pancreatic cancer and its treatment by implanted radium. Ann Surg 100:215-223, 1934
34. Pack, GT, G McNeer, Radiation treatment of pancreatic cancer. Amer J Roentgenol 40:708-714, 1938
35. Fortner, JG, GJ D'Angio, BS Hilaris, et al, Iodine 125 implantation for unresectable cancer of the pancreas. Postgrad Med 47:226-230, 1970
36. Richards, GE, Possibilities of roentgen-ray treatment in cancer of the pancreas. Amer J Roentgenol 9:150-152, 1922
37. Moertel, CG, Exocrine pancreas. In: Cancer Medicine, Holland JS, E Frei III (eds), Philadelphia, Lea and Febiger, 1973, p 1559-1590
38. Moertel, CG, DS Childs, RJ Reitemeier, et al, Combined 5-fluorouracil and supervoltage radiation therapy of locally unresectable gastrointestinal cancer. Lancet ii:865-867, 1969
39. Billingsley, JS, LG Bartholomew, DS Childs, A study of radiation therapy in carcinoma of the pancreas. Staff Mtgs Mayo Clinic 33:426-430, 1958
40. Haslam, JB, PJ Cavanaugh, SL Stroup, Radiation therapy in the treatment of irresectable adenocarcinoma of the pancreas. Cancer 32:1341-1345, 1973
41. Dobelbower, RR, Jr, KA Strubler, N Suntharalingam, Treatment of cancer of the pancreas with high-energy photons and electrons. Intl J Rad Onc 1:141-146, 1977
42. Childs, DS, CG Moertel, MA Holbrook, et al, Treatment of malignant neoplasms of the gastrointestinal tract with a combination of 5-fluorouracil and radiation. Radiol 84:843, 1965
43. Moertel, CG, DS Childs, RJ Reitemeier, et al, Combined chemotherapy and radiation therapy. In: Advanced Gastrointestinal Cancer: Clinical Management and Chemotherapy. New York, Harper and Row, 1970, p 192-204
44. Lokich, JJ, Comparative therapeutic trial of radiation with or without chemotherapy in pancreatic carcinoma. Ann Surg (in press)
45. Moertel, CG, JJ Lokich, PS Schein, et al, An evaluation of high dose radiation and combined radiation and 5-fluorouracil therapy for locally unresectable pancreatic carcinoma. Proc Amer Soc Clin Onc 17:244, 1976

46. Catterall, M, A report of three years' fast neutron therapy from the Medical Research Council's Cyclotron at Hammersmith Hospital, London. Cancer 34:91-95, 1974

47. Macdonald, JS, F Smith, R Ornitz, et al, Phase III trial of fast neutron radiation with and without 5-fluorouracil for locally advanced pancreatic and gastric adenocarcinoma. Proc Amer Soc Clin Onc 19:377, 1978

48. Castro, JR, H Schwartz, MA Freidman, et al, Conventional radiotherapy and heavy charged particle radiotherapy in the treatment of local and regional adenocarcinoma of the pancreas. Northern California Oncology Group, Protocol 3P81 (revised), 1978

49. Levin, B, WH ReMine, RE Herman, et al, Cancer of the pancreas. Amer J Surg 135:185-191, 1978

50. Carter, SK, RL Comis, Adenocarcinoma of the pancreas, prognostic variables, and criteria of response in cancer therapy: prognostic factors and criteria of response. MJ Staquet (ed), New York, Raven Press, 1975, p 237-253

51. Macdonald, JS, L Widerlite, PS Schein, Current diagnosis and management of pancreatic carcinoma. J Natl Cancer Inst 56:1093-1099, 1976

52. Macdonald, JS, L Widerlite, PS Schein, Biology, diagosis, and chemotherapeutic management of pancreatic malignancy. In: Advances in Pharmacology and Chemotherapy. Academic Press 14:107-141, 1977

53. DiMagno, EP, JR Malagelados, WF Taylor, et al, A prospective comparison of current diagnostic tests for pancreatic cancer. New Engl J Med 297:737-742, 1977

54. Hurley, JD, EH Ellison, Chemotherapy of solid cancer arising from the gastrointestinal tract. Ann Surg 152:568-582, 1960

55. Reitemeier, RJ, CG Moertel, RG Hahn, Comparative evaluation of palliation with fluorometholone (NSC-33001), 5-fluorouracil (NSC-19893), and combined fluorometholone and 5-fluorouracil in advanced gastrointestinal cancer. Cancer Chemother Rep 51:77-80, 1967

56. Moertel, CG, RJ Reitemeier, RG Hahn, Therapy with mitomycin-C in advanced gastrointestinal cancer/clinical management and chemotherapy. Moertel, CG, RJ Reitemeier (eds), New York, Harper and Row, 1969, p 168-175

57. Moertel, CG, AJ Schutl, RJ Reitemeier, et al, Therapy for gastrointestinal cancer with the nitrosoureas alone and in drug combination. Cancer Treat Rep 60:729-732, 1976

140

58. Douglass, HO, Jr, PT Levin, CG Moertel, Nitrosoureas: useful agents for treatment of advanced gastrointestinal cancer. Cancer Treat Rep 60:769-780, 1976

59. Schein, PS, RA DeLellia, CR Kahn, et al, Islet cell tumors: current concepts and management. Ann Intern Med 79:239-257, 1973

60. Dupriest, RW, M Hintington, WH Massey, et al, Streptozotocin therapy in 22 cancer patients. Cancer 35:358-367, 1974

61. Stolkinoky, DC, L Sadoff, J Braunwald, et al, Streptozotocin in the treatment of cancer. Cancer 30:61-69, 1972

62. Schein, PS, PT Lavin, CG Moertel, et al, Randomized phase II clinical trial of adriamycin in advanced measurable pancreatic carcinoma. A Gastrointestinal Tumor Study Group report. Cancer 42:19-22, 1978

63. Kaplan, RS, Phase II trial of ICRF - 159, B-deoxythioguanosine B-2 TGdR and galactitol in advanced measurable pancreatic carcinoma. A study of GITSG. Proc Amer Soc Clin Onc 19:335, 1978

64. Yunis, AA, CK Arimura, DJ Russin, Human pancreatic carcinoma (MIA PaCa^{-2}) in continuous culture: sensitivity to asparaginase. Intl J Ca 19:128-135, 1977

65. Haslam, JB, PJ Cavanaugh, SL Stroup, Radiation therapy in the treatment of irresectable adenocarcinoma of the pancreas. Cancer 32:1341-1345, 1973

66. Solom, J, M Alexander, J Steinfeld, Cyclophosphamide: a clinical study. JAMA 183:165, 1963

67. Wintrobe, M, C Huguley, Nitrogen mustard for Hodgkin's disease, lymphosarcoma, the leukemias, and other disorders. Cancer 1:634, 1948

68. Waddell, WR, Chemotherapy for carcinoma of the pancreas. Surgery 74:420-429, 1973

69. Moertel, CG, PT Lavin, An evaluation of 5-FU, nitrosoureas and lactone combinations in the therapy of upper gastrointestinal cancer. Proc Amer Soc Clin Onc 18:344, 1977

70. Buroker, T, PN Kim, L Heilbrun, V Vaitkevicius, 5-FU infusion with mitomycin-C (MMC) vs. 5-FU infusion with methyl-CCNU (ME) in the treatment of advanced upper gastrointestinal cancer. A phase III study. Proc Amer Soc Clin Onc 19:310, 1978

71. Wiggans, G, PV Woolley, JS MacDonald, et al, Phase II trial of streptozotocin mitomycin-C and 5-fluorouracil (SMF) in the treatment of advanced pancreatic cancer. Cancer 41:387-391, 1978

72. Aberhalden, RT, RM Bukowski, CW Groppe, et al, Streptozotocin (STZ) and 5-fluorouracil (5-FU) with and without mitomycin-C (MITO) in the treatment of pancreatic adenocarcinoma. Proc Amer Soc Clin Onc 18:301, 1977

73. Smith, FP, JS Macdonald, PV Woolley, et al, Phase II evaluation of FAM, 5-fluorouracil (F), Adriamycin (A) and mitomycin-C (M) in advanced pancreatic cancer (PC). Proc Amer Soc Clin Onc 20:415, 1979

CHEMOTHERAPEUTIC MANAGEMENT OF BLADDER CANCER

Donald J. Higby

Roswell Park Memorial Institute

Buffalo, New York

INTRODUCTION

Transitional cell carcinoma of the urinary bladder is one of the leading causes of cancer death in the United States. The disease is seen most commonly in older age groups and shows a preponderance for males [1]. Carcinoma of the bladder is almost certainly produced in the majority of cases by exposure to carcinogenic substances, as evidenced by the higher frequency noted in patients with urinary tract obstruction and the increased incidence in aniline dye workers and smokers [2-4].

The disease on the average tends to be rather slowly progressive as evidenced by the fact that while the mean age at diagnosis is 63, the mean age at death is 72 [1,5]. Also reflected is the fact that bladder cancer has a heterogenous course, from the solitary, slowly growing well-differentiated papillary carcinoma easily treated with fulguration, to the anaplastic tumor which metastasizes rapidly after discovery [6].

Because the disease is often slowly progressive, tends to spread locally, is amenable to surgical and radiotherapeutic management in early stages, and occurs in a population which has a high incidence of other medical disorders, the evaluation of the role of chemotherapy has been difficult. However, a number of studies indicate that reasonable chemotherapeutic palliation is possible in perhaps as many as 50% of patients with advanced disease.

INDICATIONS FOR CHEMOTHERAPY

Chemotherapy for Advanced Disease

In the patient with metastatic, recurrent, or initially inoperable disease, palliation rather than cure is usually the object of therapy. Since palliation implies relief from or prevention of symptoms and since chemotherapy known to be effective in transitional cell carcinoma of the bladder is significantly toxic and may contribute to the morbidity of the patient, the therapist obviously must deal with each patient on an individual basis, considering his general state of health, his ability to tolerate chemotherapy and the very real question as to whether his inoperable disease is presently impairing his life or causing sufficient pain to justify the contemplated treatment program. Likewise, it should be recalled in assessing these patients that radiation therapy for localized, problem-causing tumor masses should be utilized when possible in preference to chemotherapy, since toxicity is less, response is more certain, and duration of response will in all likelihood be longer (7).

Once a decision is made to employ chemotherapy, the clinician must continually reassess the patient. Administration of two cycles of an agent or combination of agents in which toxicity is produced is probably sufficient in most situations to test whether or not the tumor is sensitive to the drug regimen. In selecting a subsequent regimen, an agent previously found ineffective in that patient should not be used a second time on questionable grounds of "synergism", since the evidence for synergism of drugs in most human tumors is virtually non-existent (8). One can, however, be certain that toxicity will occur and that effective doses of the companion agent will, perforce, have to be compromised.

In the event of tumor response or in the face of progressive disease, the course of further therapeutic manipulations is clear. It is the gray area of "stable" disease in which the therapist faces serious medical and ethical treatment decisions when toxicity from the regimen significantly impairs the life of the patient. In a slowly progressive tumor, to attribute "stability" to the chemotherapy may be wishful thinking, although many clinicians would continue therapy on that supposition.

Adjuvant chemotherapy

The indications for chemotherapy are not difficult to determine in an individual patient with metastatic or inoperable disease, but the use of chemotherapy regimens for prevention of recurrence is still in question.

Jewitt correlated five year survival after total tumor resection with histologic and clinical staging (9). In patients having lesions classifiable as Stage B2 (invasion of deep muscle) or beyond, the likelihood of tumor recurrence in regional nodes or at distant sites is at least 50%. While judicious postoperative radiation therapy may reduce the likelihood of recurrence somewhat, the high incidence of local recurrence in patients treated with radiation alone (7,10) precludes advocating this routinely as an adjuvant therapy without further careful study. Chemotherapy as an adjuvant is currently in trial. At the present time, it is premature to recommend its use routinely, but in view of the predictability of recurrence in patients with more advanced stages of local disease after "curative" resection, clinicians are strongly urged to affiliate with cooperative study groups so that the participation of their patients in such studies will permit rapid assessment of the value of adjuvant chemotherapy.

CHEMOTHERAPEUTIC AGENTS USEFUL IN TRANSITIONAL CELL CARCINOMA OF THE BLADDER

Table 1

DRUGS USEFUL IN TRANSITIONAL
CELL CARCINOMA OF THE BLADDER

	Overall Reported Response Rate
Active	
Adriamycin	35%
Cis-platinum	35%
Cyclophosphamide	25-50%
5-fluorouracil	15-25%[*]
Possible Active	
Mitomycin C	10-20%
Methotrexate	+
Bleomycin	+
Hydroxyurea	+

[*]extremely wide range of reported
response rates.

[+]insufficient cases reported to estimate
response rates.

Adriamycin

Adriamycin, an antitumor antibiotic, is the single best agent currently available for transitional cell carcinoma of the bladder. Several carefully performed clinical trials suggest that the objective tumor response rate is about 35%, with an additional group of patients exhibiting subjective improvement or stable disease (21-25). Although responses are short (four to six months on the average), occasional patients will enjoy prolonged periods of clinical benefit.

Adriamycin is cardiotoxic, exhibits considerable gastrointestinal, mucosal and hematologic toxicity and also produces alopecia. Given concurrently or continuously with radiation therapy, it has been known to produce unacceptable synergistic toxicity. Also, recall reactions in sites of previous irradiation may produce serious problems.

A reasonable schedule for adriamycin alone would be 60-80 mg/M^2 given intravenously every three to four weeks. A total dose of 500 mg/M^2 should not be exceeded, as the incidence of clinically significant cardiotoxicity increases to unacceptable levels beyond that limit. The therapeutic/toxic ratio for adriamycin seems to be very narrow, and a not uncommonly encountered error in its use is to administer small, infrequent doses at the level producing no real toxicity. Conversely, a patient who does not respond to conventional doses of the agent and has minimal toxicity should be given carefully escalated doses until moderate transient marrow suppression is achieved, before concluding that the agent is ineffective. Patients with hepatic impairment sufficient to elevate bilirubin should be given adriamycin cautiously with appropriate dose adjustment.

Cis-platinum diammine dichloride

Cis-platinum is a new agent which, despite acting as an alkylating agent (26) shows no cross resistance with conventional alkylating agents in animal systems (27,28). The agent has a broad spectrum of activity in human tumors and is particularly effective in embryonal cell carcinoma of the testes (29) and ovarian carcinoma (30). Although dose-limiting toxicity is renal dysfunction when the agent is administered as an injection, much larger doses can be administered when accompanied by large fluid loads and vigorous diuresis. Under such circumstances, hematologic toxicity may become dose-limiting. In addition, the agent produces tinnitus and high frequency tone hearing loss, moderate to severe nausea and vomiting, and occasionally produces neurotoxicity (31,32) and allergic reactions (33). Like adriamycin, cis-platinum appears to have an overall response rate in excess of 30% and this may be higher in patients who have previously not been exposed to chemotherapy (34).

Cis-platinum is a difficult drug to administer and toxicity associated with the agent is exaggerated in elderly patients. To achieve appropriate plasma and tissue levels, high-dose regimens with diuresis are preferable. However, this means that the patient must have an intact cardiovascular system and normally functioning kidneys to handle the fluid load. Severe nausea, vomiting, and anorexia may also be unacceptable complications in patients already ravaged by age and cancer. Thus, while cis-platinum is an effective agent, it is not easy to use, and patients should probably be hospitalized during and after administration to assure uneventful hydration and diuresis.

An appropriate dose schedule for cis-platinum used alone would be 60-120 mg/M^2 given every four weeks, lower doses being used in older patients and patients with compromised renal function, previous prolonged aminoglycoside therapy, or previous nephrectomy. Prior to administration of the agent, and for at least six hours afterwards, the urine output should be 100 or more ml per hour. To achieve this, patients should be prehydrated with large volumes of intravenous fluid, given furosemide and/or perhaps mannitol (with larger doses). Several regimens for the administration of cis-platinum with diuresis have been published (35,36).

Cyclophosphamide

Cyclophosphamide is probably an effective single agent in bladder cancer (18,19), although there are few easily interpretable clinical trials of this agent in sufficiently large groups of patients with appropriate attention to stratification parameters and response reporting. In one study, a 38% complete and partial response rate was noted (5). On the basis of such data, the agent has been incorporated into several combination chemotherapy protocols.

Cyclophosphamide is an alkylating agent, the major toxicity of which is myelosuppression. Hemorrhagic and non-hemorrhagic sterile cystitis are occasionally serious complications seen most commonly with either prolonged continuous (daily) therapy or "megadose" infusions. Proper hydration and attention to adequate urine production should minimize this complication. Patients receiving cyclophosphamide frequently develop alopecia.

Ironically, this drug has been implicated in the genesis of bladder cancer in some patients (20) and practicing oncologists should entertain a high degree of suspicion in the patient on chronic cyclophosphamide therapy with new complaints of bladder symptomatology.

An appropriate dose schedule for this agent used alone would be 400-1000 mg/M^2 intravenously every three to four weeks.

5-fluorouracil

The status of 5-fluorouracil with respect to bladder cancer is currently in question. Several clinical trials have been reported, the majority suggesting that the agent is effective in 15-25% of patients in terms of objective regressions of disease (11-13). However, some studies have been reported showing an insignificant response rate (14-16), and in a controlled trial comparing 5-FU to placebo, no statistically significant differences were seen (17).

The drug is an antimetabolite and the mode of administration which results in maximal efficacy and minimal toxicity is not known. A reasonable schedule is 15 mg/kg/day intravenously for four to five days, followed by weekly injections in the same dose range. The drug does suppress the bone marrow, but toxicity to the gastrointestinal tract in terms of diarrhea, nausea, mucositis, etc., can be dose limiting and may become progressively more severe with increasing total cumulative doses.

Since more effective single agent therapy exists, and since the true efficacy of the drug is still in question, 5-FU should not be used alone as initial chemotherapy for bladder cancer.

Other agents

Mitomycin C (37), methotrexate (38), bleomycin (5), hydroxyurea (39) and some other agents have all been associated with objective responses in transitional cell carcinoma of the bladder. However, these agents have not been subjected to adequate trial to permit a realistic assessment of their value relative to their toxicity.

COMBINATION CHEMOTHERAPY FOR TRANSITIONAL CELL CARCINOMA OF THE BLADDER

The rationale for combination chemotherapy is well known. Given a tumor in which there is a heterogenicity of growth cycles, variably developed drug detoxification systems, different orders of membrane permeability, etc., the use of two or more effective agents with differing mechanisms of action is likely to result in the destruction of a greater amount of tumor than one agent alone. If the agents used have different toxicity patterns, their combination results in a useful increase in the therapeutic/toxic ratio.

The combinations shown in Table II are not all-inclusive, but represent recently performed studies which tend to confirm the hypothesis that multiple agents used concurrently increase response rates and have acceptable toxicity. It should be noted that since these studies consist of small numbers of patients, it cannot be definitively concluded that any of the reported combinations is superior to the best single agent given appropriately, although the results look quite promising.

In the chemotherapeutic management of patients with transitional cell carcinoma of the bladder, it is advisable to use effective combinations initially, and when these become ineffective, to use single agents. The higher response rate with combinations is associated with a longer response duration, which correlates directly with survival. In addition, patients are, as a rule, in better general condition to tolerate the additional toxicity of a combination earlier in the course of their illness.

TABLE 2

COMBINATION CHEMOTHERAPY IN TRANSITIONAL CELL CARCINOMA OF THE BLADDER

Drug & Dose	Frequency (days)	Number Evaluated	Response Rates	Reference
Adriamycin 50 mg/M^2 5-fluorouracil 500 mg/M^2	21	20	7 CR + PR 9 improved*	(40)
Adriamycin 40 mg/M^2 Cyclophosphamide 800 mg/M^2	21-28	15	8 CR + PR 4 improved*	(5)
Cis-platinum[+] Adriamycin 50 mg/M^2 5-fluorouracil 500 mg/M^2	28	17	10 CR + PR 2 improved*	(41)
Cis-platinum 1.6 mg/kg Cyclophosphamide 250-1000 mg/M^2	21-28	32	15 CR + PR 2 improved*	(42)

* 20 mg/M^2 daily for 5 days for first three cycles, then 50-75 mg/M^2 every four weeks
[+] includes "minor" responses, disease "stabilization" or "subjective" improvement

While large, well controlled group studies will eventually determine optimal combinations, it would be reasonable in the context of office practice to use a combination of adriamycin and cyclophosphamide initially, and after disease progression becomes evident, to use cis-platinum. As indicated above, the role of 5-fluorouracil is still in question and is not advocated as part of a combination at this point. On the other hand, there is no good evidence that the addition of cis-platinum to an adriamycin-cyclophosphamide combination would improve results sufficiently to justify the greatly added toxicity and the increased commitment of personnel time, hospital space, etc. required to administer that agent safely and in effective doses.

CONCLUSIONS AND PROSPECTUS

Systemic chemotherapy for advanced transitional cell carcinoma of the bladder has only recently begun to be critically examined. It appears that this disease has the same order of responsiveness as carcinoma of the breast or carcinoma of the ovary. Although substantial palliative benefit can be offered to selected patients with advanced disease using currently available drugs and combination regimens, there is need for development of more effective regimens and testing of other drugs whose efficacy in the disease is still in some question. In addition to improving chemotherapeutic regimens, exploration of the role of chemotherapy as adjuvant to primary management with surgery or radiation therapy is an urgent project. Well controlled trials, however, are necessary to determine whether a significant impact on disease recurrence can be achieved by the addition of chemotherapy to definitive surgical treatment of advanced localized disease.

The role of chemotherapy in improving the resectability of disease should also be investigated. Given the response rate and tolerable toxicity of some combination chemotherapy regimens, this may become an important part of management.

In summary, transitional cell carcinoma of the bladder which usually begins unifocally, spreads locally and regionally before systemic spread. It is usually sensitive to surgery, radiation, and chemotherapy, and should be approached at every stage of management with a true multi-disciplinary approach.

REFERENCES

1. Silverberg, E, A Halleb, Cancer statistics - 1972. Cancer 22:2, 1972

2. Cole, P, RR Manson, H Haring, et al, Smoking and cancer of the lower urinary tract. New Engl J Med 284:129, 1971

3. Cole, P, R Hoover, GH Friedell, Occupational cancer of the lower urinary tract. Cancer 29:1250, 1972

4. Hoover, R, P Cole, Temperal aspects of occupational bladder carcinogenesis. New Engl J Med 288:1040, 1973

5. Murphy, GP, Chemotherapy of bladder cancer. NY State J Med 38:1889, 1977

6. del Regato, JA, HJ Spjut, Cancer: Diagnosis, Treatment, and Prognosis. 5th edition, St. Louis, Missouri, C.V. Mosby, Co., 1977, p 637-639

7. Goffinet, DR, MJ Schreider, EJ Glatstein, et al, Bladder cancer: results of radiation therapy in 384 patients. Radiol 117:149, 1975

8. Tannock, I, Cell kinetics and chemotherapy: a critical review. Cancer Treat Rep 62:1117, 1978

9. Jewitt, HJ, Cancer of the bladder: diagnosis and staging. Cancer 32:1072, 1973

10. Wizenberg, MJ, FG Bloedorn, JD Young, et al, Radiation therapy and surgery in the treatment of carcinoma of the bladder. Amer J Roentgenol 96:113, 1966

11. Wilson, W, Chemotherapy of human solid tumors with 5-fluorouracil. Cancer 13:1230, 1960

12. Moore, G, ID Bross, R Ausman, et al, Effect of 5-fluorouracil in 389 patients with cancer. Cancer Chemother Rep 52:641, 1968

13. Glenn, J, L Hunt, J Cathem, Chemotherapy of bladder carcinoma with 5-fluorouracil. Cancer Chemother Rep 27:67, 1963

14. Ansfield, F, J Schroeder, A Carreri, Five years clinical experience with 5-fluorouracil. JAMA 181:295, 1962

15. Field, J, Fluorouracil treatment of advanced cancer in ambulatory patients. Cancer Chemother Rep 24:99, 1962

16. Weiss, A, L Jackson, R Carabasi, An evaluation of 5-fluorouracil in malignant disease. Ann Intern Med 55:731, 1961

17. Prout, GR, ID Bross, NH Slack, et al, Carcinoma of the bladder: 5-fluorouracil and the critical role of a placebo. Cancer 22:926, 1968

18. Pavone-Macaluso, M, Chemotherapy of vesical and prostatic tumors. Brit J Urol 43:701, 1971

19. Fox, M, The effect of cyclophosphamide on some urinary tract tumors. Brit J Urol 37:399, 1965

20. Wall, RL, KP Clausen, Carcinoma of the urinary bladder in patients receiving cyclophosphamide. New Engl J Med 293:271, 1975

21. Bonadonna, G, Phase I and preliminary Phase II evaluation of adriamycin. Cancer Res 30:2752, 1970

22. Tan, C, E Etcubanas, N Wollner, et al, Adriamycin-an antitumor antibiotic in the treatment of neoplastic diseases. Cancer 32:9, 1973

23. Middleman, E, J Luce, E Frei, Clinical trials with adriamycin. Cancer 28:844, 1971

24. O'Bryan, RM, Phase II evaluation of adriamycin in human neoplasia. Cancer 32:1, 1973

25. Weinstein, SH, JD Schmidt, Doxorubicin chemotherapy in advanced transitional cell carcinoma. Urology 8:336, 1976

26. Rosenberg, B, L Van Camp, JE Trosko, et al, Platinum compounds: a new class of potent antitumor agents. Nature 222:385, 1969

27. Sirica, A, JM Venditti, I Kline, Enhanced survival response of L-1210 leukemic mice to a single combination treatment with cis-platinum (II) diammine dichloride plus cyclophosphamide. Proc Amer Assoc Cancer Res 12:4, 1971

28. Speer, RJ, S Lapis, H Ridgeway, et al, Cis-platinum diamminodichloride in combination therapy of leukemia L-1210. Wadley Med Bull 1:103, 1971

29. Higby, DJ, HJ Wallace, Jr, D Albert, JF Holland, A phase I study showing responses in testicular and other tumors. Cancer 33:1219, 1974

30. Wiltshaw, E, T Kroner, Phase II study of cis-dichlorodiammineplatinum in advanced adenocarcinoma of the ovary. Cancer Treat Rep 60:55, 1976

31. Bruckner, HW, CJ Cohen, B Kabakow, et al, Combination chemotherapy of ovarian carcinoma with platinum: improved therapeutic index. Proc Amer Assoc Cancer Res 18:339, 1977

32. Ostrow, S, D Hahn, P Wiernik, et al, Ophthalmologic toxicity after cis-dichlorodiammine-platinum therapy. Cancer Treat Rep 62:1591, 1978

33. Kahn, A, JM Hill, W Grater, et al, Atopic hypersensitivity to cis-dichlorodiammineplatinum and other platinum complexes. Cancer Res 35:2766, 1975

34. Yagoda, A, R Watson, JC Gonzalez-Vitale, Cis-dichlorodiammineplatinum in advanced bladder cancer. Cancer Treat Rep 60:917, 1976

152

35. Hayes, D, E, Cvitkovic, R Goldberg, et al, Amelioration of renal toxicity of high dose cis-platinum diammine dichloride by mannitol induced diuresis. Proc Amer Assoc Cancer Res 17:109, 1976

36. Merrin, C, A new method to prevent toxicity with high doses of cis-diammine platinum. Proc Amer Assoc Cancer Res 17:243, 1976

37. Early, K, EG Elias, A Mittelman, et al, Mitomycin C in the treatment of metastatic transitional cell carcinoma of the urinary bladder. Cancer 31:1150, 1973

38. Altman, CC, NJ McCague, AC Ripepi, The use of methotrexate in advanced carcinoma of the bladder. J Urol 108:271, 1972

39. Howe, C, M Samuels, Phase II studies of hydroxyurea in adults: urologic and gynecologic neoplasms. Cancer Chemother Rep 40:47, 1964

40. Cross, RJ, GP Yorkshire, Treatment of advanced bladder cancer with adriamycin and fluorouracil. Brit J Urol 48:605, 1976

41. Williams, SD, RJ Rohn, JP Donahue, et al, Chemotherapy of bladder cancer with cis-diammine dichloroplatinum, adriamycin, and 5-fluorouracil. Proc Amer Assoc Cancer Res 19:316, 1978

42. Yagoda, A, R Watson, N Kemeny, et al, Diammine dichloride platinum II and cyclophosphamide in the treatment of advanced urothelial cancer. Cancer 41:2121, 1978

MAMMOGRAPHY

Erlinda S. McCrea, M.D.
Department of Radiology
University of Maryland Hospital
Baltimore, Maryland

HISTORICAL PERSPECTIVE

Mammography is the roentgenologic examination of the breast. Today it has a definite role in the screening, localization and diagnosis of breast cancer. The purpose of this paper is to review the indications for mammography, the current doses and risks of various techniques, and the mammographic patterns of breast cancer and its differential diagnosis. We will also look into the advantages of needle localization by mammography and the use of specimen radiography.

Salomon (1), a German surgeon, first used roentgenography in 1913 to study gross mastectomy specimens. In 1930, Warren (2), an American radiologist, reported on the clinical use of mammography. Over the years since then interest in mammography has waxed and waned, concomitant with changing and improving techniques, the changing status of breast cancer management and results, eventually resulting in better definition of the precise role of mammography in breast cancer. In 1956, Egan developed a high milliamperage, low kilovoltage, long exposure-time technique at the M.D. Anderson Hospital, using industrial grade film (Kodak M), which resulted in a simple and reproducible mammographic technique with good detail (3). Improvements in this technique, as well as the evolution of other plain film mammographic techniques continue, resulting in better imaging of breast tissue and pathology. A further refinement in technique came about when John Wolfe (4) and John Martin (5) pioneered the xerographic method which did not come into general use until 1972. Xeroradiography is the production of an image utilizing a photoconductive surface (a selenium-coated plate contained in a cassette), electrostatic charges and x-rays. A pigmented developing powder (blue toner) produces a permanent image on a sheet of plastic-coated paper for viewing and storage. Xerography has good resolution capabilities and has the unique property of edge enhancement or "edge effect". The contrast between differences in tissue density is greatly enhanced due to the fact that the toner-attracting fields from the electrostatic image are strongest at such boundaries. As a result, it is considered by many to be the optimal technique for mammography (6).

153

RADIATION DOSAGE

Technique and Dose

With increasing concern about dosages and competition from various manufacturers to produce lower dose imaging systems, the emphasis on optimal mammographic image quality has evolved into the problem of retaining acceptable image quality while striving for lower doses. Early studies in the 1960's showed exposure doses at skin surfaces as high as 4 to 8 roentgens. Subsequent improvement in techniques have lowered the doses to the current doses of 0.4 to 1 roentgen per exposure per breast. Continued improvements without compromising image quality may hopefully achieve surface doses as low as 100 milliroentgens per exposure. The current dose per exposure at the skin surface at our institution is 450 milliroentgens. A complete mammographic study entails a craniocaudad and a lateral view, with an axillary view being optional. Following calculations for conversion into rads and amount of filtration used, the absorbed dose per study equals 80 to 100 millirads at the midplane of the breast.

Dose and Complications

Since mammography is a diagnostic and screening tool, the question of radiation-induced complications such as cancer of the breast must be addressed. The precise hazard of radiation to the breast is still speculative. Data on this subject have been derived from several sources: animals exhibiting spontaneous breast neoplasm after various radiation dosages, backward extrapolations made from individuals exposed at Hiroshima, females treated with radiation for postpartum mastitis, women irradiated for pulmonary tuberculosis using multiple fluoroscopic examinations, etc. These data suggest a linear extrapolation to low dosages, but this is too simple an explanation when multiple factors, many unknown, are involved in breast neoplasia. Thus, the issue remains unsettled. One positive note can be made in this regard. Mammography has been used for well over 20 years, with much greater doses used in the early years. Yet there is not one proven case of breast cancer associated with mammography (7).

Let us look at the issue in another way. The age-adjusted incidence for breast cancer in American women is 70/1000/year or 7%. Utilizing a single low-dose mammographic examination, delivery of one rad per breast increases the lifetime risk of developing breast cancer from 7% to 7.07%. In other words, it would take 100 mammographic examinations of each breast to change the risk from 70/1000/year to 70.7/1000/year (7). Therefore, when mammography is indicated, the risk of possible complications should not deter one from using the examination.

INDICATIONS FOR MAMMOGRAPHY

Indications for mammography have varied over the years. It was initially used to confirm a clinically palpable lesion and to help with staging (e.g., presence or absence of positive axillary lymph nodes), while its current role is to detect occult or nonpalpable lesions. Screening programs such as the Health Insurance Plan of Greater New York (HIP) and the ongoing Breast Cancer Detection Demonstration Projects (BCDDP) attest to the fact that mammography is of proven value (8) in at least certain portions of the population.

Indications for Initial Mammography

1. Preoperative evaluation - Both breasts should be examined, not only to confirm the clinically palpable lesion but to evaluate the opposite breast since bilateral and simultaneous cancers occur in 1.7 to 2% of cases, frequently revealing different histologic types within the same breast (9,10).
2. High risk patients
    a. Nulliparity
    b. Late parity (28 years or later) (11)
    c. History of breast cancer in immediate family, e.g. sister, mother
    d. Prior benign breast surgery - including papillomatosis, ductal thickening or hyperplasia and cystic disease (9)
3. Palpable mass or masses - whether biopsy is contemplated or not
4. Large, difficult-to-examine breasts
5. Other complaints or physical findings such as ulceration, discharge, dimpling, nipple retraction or skin thickening
6. Metastases with an unidentified primary lesion - an occult breast cancer may be present

Indications for Serial Studies

1. Prior breast cancer - Examination of the opposite breast is recommended 6 months after surgery for breast cancer and yearly therafter. Up to 16% of these patients will eventually develop a second primary in the opposite breast, with half of these occurring within 6 years following mastectomy (12).
2. Strong family history of breast cancer
3. Breast dysplasia, especially those conditions associated with a high risk for development of cancer
4. Previous equivocal mammogram
5. Previous mammoplasty or subcutaneous mastectomy with implant (9)

Mammography for screening

Screening has been advocated for asymptomatic women over 50 years of age (9,11,13). Occult cancers found by mammography are potentially curable, since results of axillary lymph-node biopsy have been negative in 77% of these patients (9). One-third of these lesions would have been missed if only history and physical examination had been relied upon (13).

Mammography is most accurate in women 50 years of age and older because of fatty replacement of breast tissue following menopause, making masses more readily discernible radiologically. Mammography is less helpful in women under 35 years of age for two reasons: premenopausal breast tissue shows a dense mammographic pattern which tends to obscure underlying disease, and breast cancer has a much lower incidence in women of this age group (9).

According to recent BCDDP reports (8,13), mammography is superior to physical examination in detecting occult or minimal cancers (less than 1 cm. in diameter):

mammography 95%

physical examination 33%

Therefore, mammography should be employed whenever a mass is palpable or any of the high-risk factors exist. Screening programs have been successful in detecting highly localized disease with over a third of detectable lesions being noninfiltrating or infiltrating but less than 1 cm. in size and at least 70% having negative axillary nodes (13).

MAMMOGRAPHIC FEATURES OF BREAST CANCER

The major features of breast cancer are: mass, tumor calcifications and duct pattern.

Mass

Approximately 80 to 90% of cancers are evident by their mass density (4). The appearance is variable, ranging from an obvious spiculated scirrhous carcinoma (figure 1) to a very subtle asymmetric "increased density" in a limited area in one breast (figure 2). Other forms include nodular, lobulated, smooth, and diffuse as is seen in inflammatory carcinoma (figure 3).

The spiculation and irregularity of scirrhous tumors reflect the locally aggressive, infiltrating character of the cancer into the surrounding tissues. Highly infiltrative carcinomas tend to feel much larger upon clinical examination than their mammographic dimensions suggest due to the surrounding desmo-plastic reaction, while well-circumscribed tumors tend to feel almost the same size as their mammographic images appear (14).

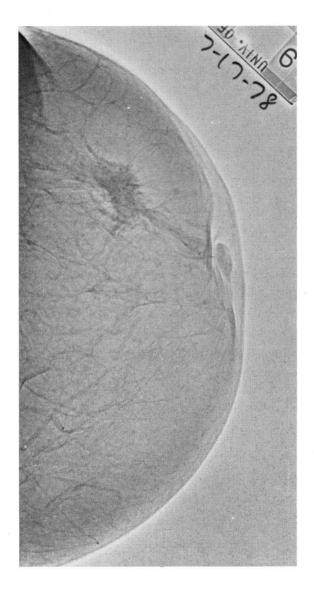

Figure 1: Scirrhous cancer showing spiculated margins and microcalcifications.

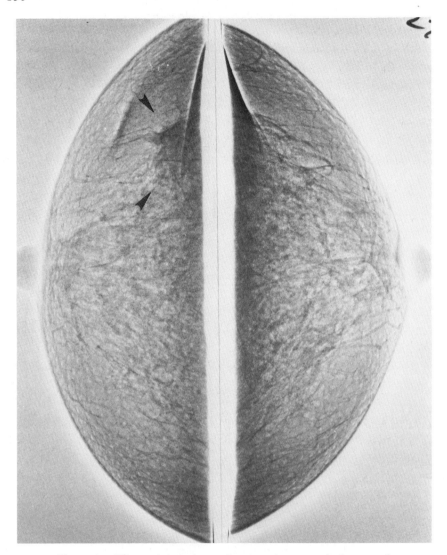

Figure 2: Bilateral ductal prominence. Asymmetric increased density in juxtathoracic region of outer quadrant, with slightly irregular margins (arrows). Proven intraductal carcinoma.

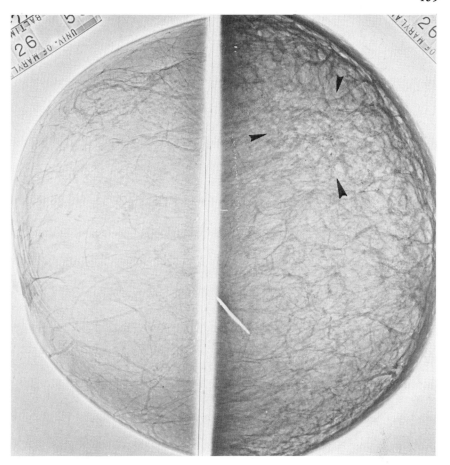

Figure 3: Diffuse increased density with marked skin thickening. Cluster of calcifications with associated ill-defined mass density (arrows). Typical inflammatory carcinoma.

160

Examples of well-circumscribed carcinomas include colloid (mucinous) carcinoma (figure 4), tubular carcinoma and medullary carcinoma which have a slower growth and a more favorable prognosis.

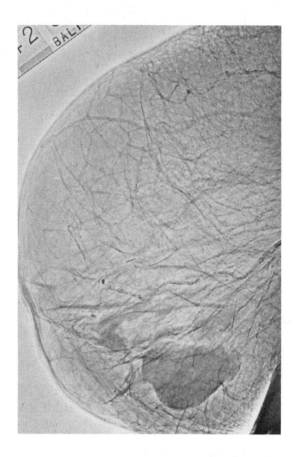

Figure 4: Smooth, somewhat lobulated mass suggesting benign lesion proved to be mucinous carcinoma.

In contrast to the infiltrative character of most carcinomas, the great majority of benign masses such as cysts and fibroadenomas appear pathologically and mammographically to be more circumscribed and well delineated. However, the occasionally well-defined tumors such as medullary, colloid and intracystic carcinomas can resemble benign lesions. It is, therefore, wise to perform excisional biopsy of solitary masses, especially in women who are at risk for cancer, regardless of the clinical or mammographic features (14).

Calcifications

Calcific deposits are seen in both benign and malignant disease. The importance of those associated with breast cancer cannot be underestimated. They can be identified in as many as 40% of cancers on xerographs and may also provide the only indication of malignancy in 16% of cases, especially the comedocarcinoma variety (10). These calcific deposits are small (0.1 to 2 mm.), round, rod-shaped or lace-like and usually have irregular margins. They are usually clustered with 15 to 20 deposits (figure 5) but can be as few as 2 or 3. They may be grouped together within the mass or widely separated as in comedocarcinoma (4).

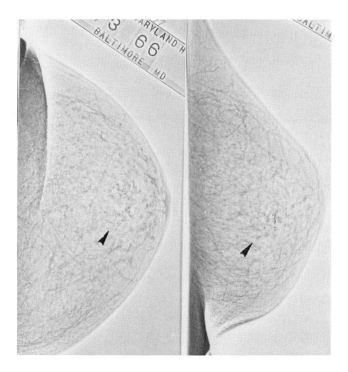

Figure 5: Cluster of calcifications posterior and inferior to nipple without associated mass was proved intraductal cancer (arrows).

Duct Patterns

An asymmetrical collection of ducts in one breast without a similar change in the opposite breast may be a clue to the presence of a carcinoma. Occasionally, segmental prominence is another ductal pattern that may be observed mammographically (10). This finding may be seen in 18% of cases. Recently ductal patterns and density of the breast have been suggested as being indicative and prognostic of malignant and premalignant lesions and this will be discussed by Wolfe elsewhere in this publication.

DIFFERENTIAL DIAGNOSIS OF BREAST CANCER ON MAMMOGRAPHY

Cysts

These result from localized duct distension, and as further cystic fluid accumulates, the distended cyst wall creates a smooth, sharp border. This can be confirmed by aspiration.

Fibroadenoma

This is the commonest, solid, benign tumor of the breast. Fibroadenomas (figure 6) can grow rapidly during adolescence, pregnancy or menopause. They can be single or multiple. With advancing age, these tumors may degenerate and undergo coarse calcification.

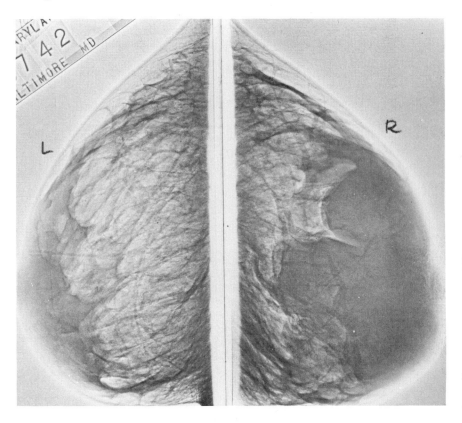

Figure 6: Multiple fibroadenomas of varying sizes in a 17 year old female.

Sclerosing adenosis

This is the most common benign disorder which can be incorrectly diagnosed as malignant by the mammographer. It usually appears as an ill-defined, irregular or nodular process containing small flecks or calcific deposits. The process is usually bilateral and symmetrical, but can be asymmetric. When this situation occurs, particularly when the cluster of calcifications simulates that of carcinoma, biopsy is mandatory to exclude cancer (14).

Breast abscess

This may cause diffuse thickening of the skin but is more often localized. Frequently, this disorder may be differentiated from cancer only by biopsy.

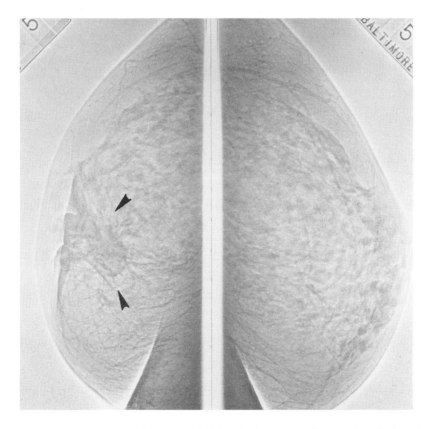

Figure 7: Retro-areolar mass with nipple retraction and spiculated margins suspicious for cancer but proved to be fat necrosis on biopsy (arrows).

Fat necrosis

This lesion is a nonsuppurative process that occurs most often in the fatty, large breasts of middle-aged women and usually results from trauma. The features of fat necrosis are variable and occasionally may simulate those of carcinoma, with severe desmoplastic reaction, spiculation and thickening and retraction of overlying skin (figure 7 - compare with figure 8).

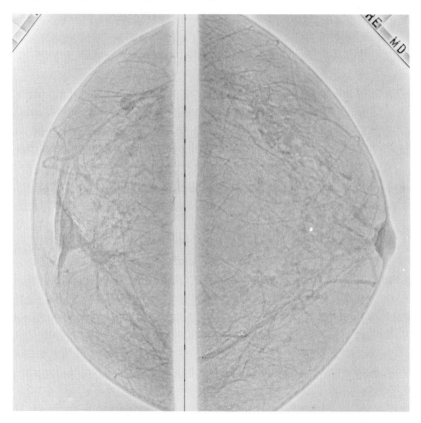

Figure 8: Retro-areolar mass with nipple retraction, irregular margins and calcifications was proven intraductal carcinoma (see Figure 6).

Metastatic disease to the breast

These lesions are unusual with only 152 reported cases in the world literature (15). They tend to be painless, discrete lumps that are generally small and single at the time of discovery. The most common primary sites are: melanoma, lung cancer (especially the oat cell variety), stomach, ovaries, kidneys and cervix. Lymphoma and leukemia are another occasional source.

Biopsy scars

Biopsy scars can create confusion especially when a stellate scar forms, simulating carcinoma (figure 9). History and physical examination would be helpful when in doubt.

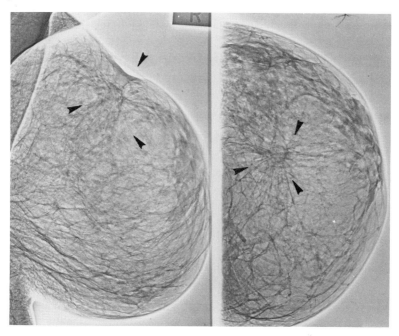

Figure 9: Upper outer quadrant mass (arrows) with irregular, spiculated margins and skin retraction suggest cancer. Proven biopsy scar.

MAMMOGRAPHIC NEEDLE LOCALIZATION

As mammographic techniques improve, we are detecting more and more breast lesions which are radiographically suspicious for carcinoma but too small to be clinically palpable. Biopsy of these clinically occult lesions can be difficult. Preoperative mammograms are not reliable for precise location for biopsy, since the location of the lesion on the mammogram may differ greatly from its actual location in the breast when the patient is on the operating table (16,17). This may occur because the breast is a pliable organ; during mammography the breast is compressed away from the chest wall whereas during surgery it is flattened on the chest wall and the patient is supine. As a consequence, a "blind" open biopsy of an occult lesion may completely miss the lesion, requiring extension of the biopsy, prolonged anesthesia time and increased postsurgical scarring and deformity (18). Mammographic needle localization, as the current technique has evolved, has proved to be the definitive method in precise localization for biopsy of nonpalpable breast lesions. The goal is the resection of the smallest possible amount of breast tissue while ensuring that the biopsy contains the suspicious area. A variety of mammographic localization procedures have been described in the literature, all of which are highly accurate (16-22). So far, no complications have been reported. The basic principle in all the described methods is the percutaneous insertion of a needle into the breast tissue in as close proximity as is possible to the suspicious area, followed by radiographic verification of the satisfactory needle position (figure 10). The needle may be left in place after

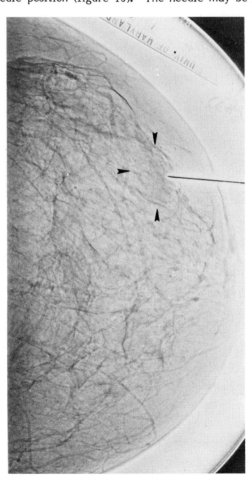

Figure 10: Nonpalpable mass in outer quadrant localized with needle prior to surgical biopsy. Proven fibrocystic disease with ductal hyperplasia (arrows).

being snugly taped to prevent inadvertent removal while the patient is taken to the surgical suite. The surgeon then uses the needle as a visual guide to surgical biopsy. Another approach is to inject dye into the lesion, leaving dye in the needle tract. The dye tract is then used for visual guidance at biopsy. Biopsy must be done within 30 minutes to one hour following this maneuver to prevent significant diffusion of the dye into the surrounding tissues. These procedures naturally entail close communication and cooperation between the radiologist, the surgeon and the pathologist (14).

SPECIMEN RADIOGRAPHY

Specimen radiography can be done on the surgical specimen, either following prior needle localization or "blind" excisional biopsy of a lesion. This is done to confirm the removal of the suspicious lesion and is particularly helpful when calcifications are present. This procedure also requires close cooperation between the mammographer, the surgeon and the pathologist to ensure the rapid transit of specimens and less extensive surgical procedures.

SUMMARY

Breast carcinoma continues to be a leading cause of morbidity and mortality in women. Combined physical examination and mammography have proven to be greatly effective in detecting early breast cancer. An improved salvage rate does occur following discovery by mammography alone (23). The usefulness of mammography is directly proportional to the quality of the procedure.

Screening programs such as those conducted by BCDDP in its 29 cancer screening centers have proven the value of the detection of minimal cancers, which comprise over a third of the cancers discovered. Mammography is the primary means of detecting these cancers, especially in women over 50 years of age and in women whose physical examination is less reliable (23).

Recent reports on low-dose plain film mammographic techniques and xerographic methods have lowered the surface exposure doses and consequent midplane absorbed doses in the breast to less than 1 rad per exposure per breast (24,25). The only controlled study on the risk-benefit analyses of mammography was in the HIP study, which was conducted in 1963. These findings may not be applicable to today's methods since they were based on older and higher-dose techniques. Bailar (26) and Breslow (27) have suggested that the radiation risks of screening mammography may equal or exceed its benefits. However, they have based their analyses on the HIP study. No allowance was made for the differences in x-ray energies and patient age of the high-dose exposure situations

(Hiroshima victims, multi-fluoroscopic examinations of the chest, etc), as compared with conventional mammography where they are continually being monitored to optimize image quality while keeping low-dose exposure rates.

In view of these facts, the routine use of mammography is felt to be very beneficial in certain age groups and certainly in high risk patients. There is also an evolving body of evidence which suggests that mammographic parenchymal patterns are helpful in identifying the woman at risk for developing breast cancer.

REFERENCES

1. Salomon, A, Beitrage zur pathologie und klinik des mammarkaarzinoms. Arch KLIN Chir 101:573-668, 1913

2. Warren SL, Roetgenologic study of the breast. Amer J Roentgen 24:113-124, 1930

3. Egan, RL, Experience with mammography in a tumor institution: Evaluation of 1000 studies. Radio 75:894-900, 1960

4. Wolfe, JN, Xerography of the Breast. Radio 91:231-240, 1968

5. Martin JE, Xeromammography - An improved diagnostic method: Review of 250 biopsied cases. Amer J Roentgen 117:90-96, 1973

6. Wolfe, JN, Xeroradiography of the Breast. 1st ed. Springfield, C. C. Thomas, 1972

7. Sickles, EA, Benefits and risks of screening mammography. West J Med 126:70-71, 1977

8. BCDDP, Preliminary draft report of epidemiology-biostatistics subgroup of the working group to review NCI/ACS BCDDP, Aug 8, 1977

9. Sadowsky, NL, L Kalisher, G White, and JT Ferrucci, Jr, Radiologic detection of breast cancer - Review and Recommendations. New Engl J Med 294:370-373, 1976

10. Wolfe, JN, Analysis of 462 breast carcinomas. Amer J Roentgen 121:846-853, 1974

11. Frankl, G and M Ackerman, Risk factors and occult breast cancer in young women. Amer J Roentgen 132:427-428, 1979

12. Robbins, GF and JW Berg, Bilateral primary breast cancers: A prospective clinicopathologic study. Cancer 17:1501-1527, 1964

13. BCDDP, Report of working group to review BCDDP, Sept 6, 1977

14. Gold, RH, CK Montgomery, and ON Rambo, Significance of Margination of benign and malignant infiltrative mammary lesions: Roentgenographic pathologic correlation. Amer J Roentgen 118:881-894, 1973

15. Toombs, BD and L Kalisher, Metastatic disease to the breast: Clinical, pathologic and radiologic features. Amer J Roentgen 129:673-676, 1977

16. Dodd, GD, Preoperative radiographic localization of nonpalpable lesions, In: Early Breast Cancer, Detection and Treatment, Gallagher, HS (ed.), New York, Wiley, 151-153, 1975

17. Libshitz, HI, SA Feig, and S Fetouh, Needle localization of nonpalpable breast lesions. Radio 121:557-560, 1976

18. Bolmgren, J, B Jacobson, and B Nordenstrom, Stereotaxic instrument for needle biopsy of the mamma. Amer J Roentgen 129:121-125, 1977

19. Hall, FM and HA Frank, Preoperative localization of nonpalpable breast lesions. Amer J Roentgen 132:101-105, 1979

20. Egan, JF, CB Sayler, and MJ Goodman, A technique for localizing occult breast lesions. Cancer 26:32-37, 1976

21. Horns, JW and RD Arndt, Percutaneous spot localization of nonpalpable breast lesions. Amer J Roentgen 127:253-256, 1976

22. Kalisher, L, An improved needle for localization for nonpalpable lesions. Radio 128:815-817, 1978

23. Egan, RL, Metamorphosis of breast cancer. South Med J 71:1325-1330, 1978

24. Change, CHJ, JL Sibala, NL Martin, and RC Riley, Film mammography: New low radiation technology. Radio 121:215-217, 1978

25. Van De Riet, WG and JN Wolfe, Dose reduction in xeroradiography of the breast. Amer J Roentgen 128:821-823, 1977

26. Bailar, JC III, Mammography: A contrary view. Ann Intern Med 84:77-84, 1976

27. Breslow, L, NCI working group on gross and net benefits of mammography in mass screening for the detection of breast cancer. Mar 8, 1977

BREAST PARENCHYMAL PATTERNS ON MAMMOGRAPHY
AND THEIR RELATIONSHIP TO CARCINOMA

John N. Wolfe

Hutzel Hospital

Detroit, Michigan

INTRODUCTION

This presentation concerns itself with the problem of identifying the woman at risk for developing breast cancer by the radiographic appearance of the breast parenchyma.

It is likely that the radiologist is most qualified to identify women at risk for developing breast cancer. Work began at Hutzel Hospital in 1964 on breast parenchymal patterns and their relationship to carcinoma (1,2). It was noted, in this very early work, that a prominent duct pattern often accompanied a carcinoma, whether it be a palpable or occult neoplasm. This relationship of a prominent duct pattern with carcinoma led one to believe that perhaps the presence of a prominent duct pattern in the absence of identifiable abnormalities suggestive of carcinoma would indicate that the patient was more likely to develop the disease sometime later in life.

Several studies have been done at Hutzel Hospital, testing the hypothesis that breast parenchymal patterns are effective indicators of risk, and in the two papers published thus far, that would appear to be so (3,4). Other investigators have looked at this concept. Although some have not found it an effective indicator of risk, at least in the long term (5,6), the majority of opinion is that breast parenchymal patterns do provide a relatively good index of risk for developing breast carcinoma (7,8,9).

Two studies have been done at Hutzel Hospital evaluating breast parenchymal patterns for delineating a group of women most likely to develop breast carcinoma (3,4). The method was relatively simple. The mammograms of a large number of patients were reviewed without knowledge of whether or not the patient had a breast cancer, or her age or her status as to the usual historical risk factors, such as parity and family history. Some of the classified cases had been examined by conventional film mammography and others by xeroradiography.

172

Based on the experience of the early work at Hutzel Hospital and continued observations, four classifications were developed. It is likely that the classification system can be refined further, but the simple division of patients into one of four groups appeared to be effective. The classifications are as follows:

N1 The breast was composed almost solely of fat without demonstrable prominent ducts (figure 1)

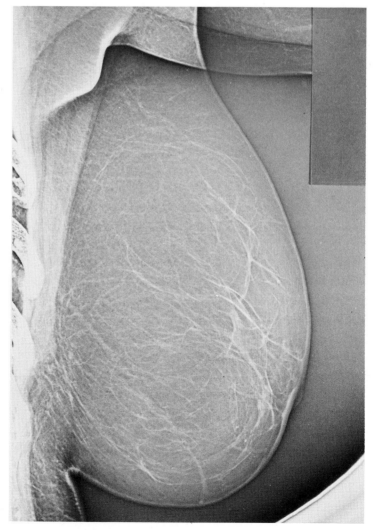

Figure 1: N1—The breast is composed almost solely of fat with a few trabeculae. No areas of dysplasia or prominent ducts can be identified.

P1 Prominent ducts were observed, but they occupied less than one-fourth of the breast (figure 2).

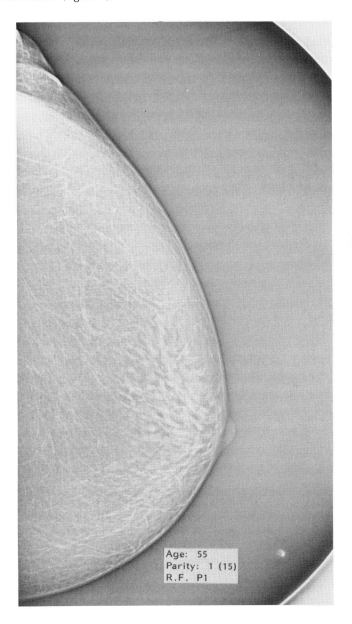

Figure 2: P1--The breast is composed almost solely of fat with the exception of the definite cordlike and nodular densities seen in the subareolar area. The degree of involvement is judged to be less than one-fourth of the breast parenchyma.

174

P2   The breast was involved with prominent ducts to a degree greater than one fourth (figure 3).

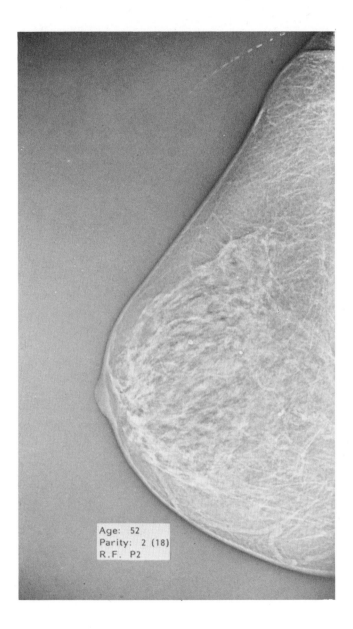

Figure 3: P2--There is a very definite cordlike and nodular appearance to almost all of the breast. This represents severe involvement with a prominent duct pattern.

DY The breast contained sheetlike areas of increased density which radiographically are termed dysplasia and correlates quite well with what the pathologist will identify as mammary dysplasia (figure 4).

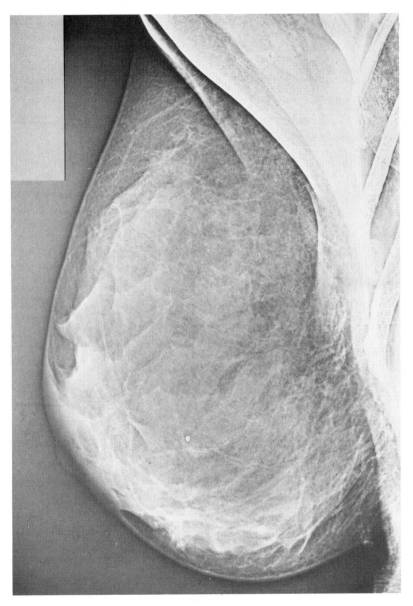

Figure 4: DY—The parenchyma is composed of sheetlike areas of increased density without the nodularity or linearity as associated with a prominent duct pattern. it represents dysplastic change and is classified as DY.

CORRELATION OF CLASSIFICATION AND CANCER

Following the classification of a relatively large number of cases, the names of the patients were submitted to the local Tumor Registry and it was searched to find which patients developed or had a breast carcinoma. Some of the women were traced by direct mailing asking them whether they had had a breast carcinoma, and if so, at what institution the surgery was performed and the date.

The object of the study and the classification system was to identify incident breast cancers and it should be stressed that it was not a study of prevalent breast cancers. As will be seen later, the distribution of parenchymal patterns between these two groups was different, prevalent versus incident, but the classification nevertheless was significant in both.

The following qualifications were necessary for inclusion into the study. The initial radiographic report must have been negative for carcinoma of the breast. Arbitrarily, any patient who had histologic proof of a breast carcinoma during an interval from the initial examination to the proof of the existence of a breast neoplasm within six months was excluded from the study. It was thought likely that these were merely prevalent breast cancers which escaped detection by the radiographic examination. There has been no study to affirm that the six-month interval was correct. Some cutoff point, however, had to be established and this seemed reasonable.

Table 1 presents the combined data from these first two studies. One should note there is a stepwise incidence of breast carcinoma occurring in the four groups, the lowest in N1 and the highest in DY, with P1 and P2 in between. It was concluded, therefore, that an assessment of the breast parenchymal pattern was a valuable aide in identifying women at risk.

Table 1

STUDIES 1967-1972

Class	Cases #	Cases %	Carcinomas #	Carcinomas %	Incidence %
N1	2751	38.13	4	5.26	0.14
P1	1820	25.22	7	9.21	0.38
P2	1948	27.00	34	44.73	1.74
DY	695	9.63	31	40.78	3.22
Total	7214	99.98	76	99.98	1.05

PREVALENT VERSUS INCIDENT CARCINOMAS

Distinction

It is important to distinguish between prevalent and incident breast carcinomas. For some this distinction may be difficult to comprehend. To illustrate the distinction, if we examined a large population such as ten thousand women aged 35 and over on one day, whether they were symptomatic or asymptomatic, we would expect to find at most about ten breast cancers per 1000 women examined. If we examined this closed group precisely one year later, we would expect the pickup rate to drop to approximately five breast carcinomas per 1000 women examined. If we continued to examine them at yearly intervals, there would be a progressive drop in the rate of pickup of breast carcinomas and one would think it would eventually stabilize to about two per thousand after three or four yearly studies. It is this plateau in the number of breast carcinomas which is regarded as incidence.

To illustrate the difference in classification between prevalent and incident carcinomas, a study was undertaken to compare what were considered incident carcinomas and prevalent carcinomas. We found a difference in the risk classifications between these two groups (10).

The prevalent carcinomas were obtained from the files of Hutzel Hospital. All patients with carcinoma over a two-year period who had had a preoperative xeroradiograph of the breast were identified. They had been classified prior to surgery. As a matching group, a consecutive number of incident carcinomas found on interval follow-up were compared. The results of this study can be seen in table 2. The important figure is the distribution of the cases among the various risk groups. One must recognize that the prevalent carcinomas were drawn from an unlimited population. The incident carcinomas were drawn from a closed population, the requirement being they must have had a negative mammogram at least six months prior to the histologic proof of carcinoma.

Table 2

RISK CLASSIFICATION

	Total	N1		P1		P2		DY	
	#	#	%	#	%	#	%	#	%
Hutzel Cases (Prevalent)	118	3	2.54	32	27.12	67	56.78	16	13.56
Interval Cases (Incident)	169	2	1.18	12	7.10	99	58.57	56	33.13

Percentages are rounded to the nearest hundredth.

Correlation of risk factors and incident carcinoma

If one combines the N1 and P1 as relatively low-risk groups and the P2 and DY as higher risk groups, we note on the one hand (prevalent) a distribution of approximately 30 percent/70 percent low risk/high risk. This can be contrasted with the 8.28 percent/91.70 percent for the incident carcinomas. One could make a conclusion based on these data that there is a propensity of incident breast carcinomas to develop in the P2-DY group (high risk) after an initial negative examination.

One might argue that the incident breast carcinomas are merely missed carcinomas. Certainly no one knows when a breast carcinoma actually begins. It is known, however, that the doubling time for the average breast carcinoma is in the realm of 120 days. One can estimate, therefore, that if on the initial radiographic study a 0.5 cm. carcinoma were present and not observed that by six months the carcinoma would be 2 cm. in size and by nine months it would be 4 cm. It is recognized, however, that various individual carcinomas of the breast grow more quickly than others, and that the numbers for doubling time given here are averages for all carcinomas, irrespective of their type. Thus, an important fact to establish is the time interval between the initial radiographic study and the histologic proof of the incident breast carcinoma. This was not short--the average for this group of patients was approximately four years and the median, three years (table 3).

Table 3

TIME BETWEEN FIRST EXAM AND
PROOF OF CARCINOMA

169 Cases

Average	50.6 months
Median	35.0 months

Further evidence that these were not merely missed carcinomas of the breast can be gained by regarding the status of the axillary lymph nodes at the time of surgery and contrasting the two groups. One would think that if these were merely missed breast carcinomas on the initial study, when they were proven there would be a greater degree of lymph node involvement with metastases than in the prevalent group, and this is not the case. As one regards table 4, one should note that there is not a great deal of difference in the number of patients with positive axillary nodes between the two groups and the slightly more favorable number for the incident carcinomas is not statistically significant.

Table 4

AXILLARY NODE STATUS

	Total		Neg Nodes		Pos Nodes	
	#	%	#	%	#	%
Hutzel	124	100	78	62.9	46	37.1
Interval	144	100	99	68.8	45	31.2

An inspection of table 5, however, reveals a number which is statistically significant. If we further analyze the patients with positive axillary lymph nodes, we find that a greater number of patients with prevalent carcinomas have more than one node positive, compared to the patients with incident carcinomas, and this comparison is statistically significant. It is concluded, therefore, that the incident carcinomas are not missed carcinomas in the usual sense, but rather are, likely, composed primarily of truly incident carcinomas. These are the true target of any screening study.

Table 5

EXTENT OF AXILLARY METASTASIS

	Total		1+		> 1+	
	#	%	#	%	#	%
Hutzel	46	100	5	10.9	41	89.1
Interval	45	100	14	31.0	31	69.0

P < 0.05

CORRELATION OF PARENCHYMAL PATTERNS WITH HISTOPATHOLOGY

Preliminary correlative studies on the histologic counterpart of the various risk patterns reveals good agreement between the radiographic indices of risk and those associated with histopathology (11). This author has been fortunate to work closely with Dr. S. Robert Wellings of the University of California at Davis. Dr. Wellings has had long experience in the study of the histopathology of the breast (12,13,14). The first published material on this work is the result of Dr. Wellings' reviewing a considerable number of consecutive biopsies done at

Table 6

CORRELATION BETWEEN HISTOPATHOLOGICAL GRADE AND
XERORADIOGRAPHIC RISK FACTOR

XR Risk Factor	# of Tumors Expected Per 1,000 Patients in 3 Yr.	# of Cases	Median Age (yr.)	Age Range (yr.)	Mean of Highest Wellings Grade	Mean ALA Score	Mean of Highest Black Grade
N1	1.4	27	43	31-76	0.52	0.85	1.30
P1	5.2	37	57	31-78	1.27	5.57	1.68
P2	19.6	44	49	38-70	2.20	16.13	2.43
DY	52.2	35	46	33-70	3.03	25.43	3.11

Hutzel Hospital without the knowledge of the radiographic risk classification. He graded the cases also by the method of Black, et al (15). As one inspects table 6, one can see that the N1-radiographic-type breast correlates very well with what Dr. Wellings regards, based on histologic appearance, as a breast at exceedingly low risk for developing breast carcinoma. He, too, found a stepwise progression of the relative risk which correlates very well with the radiographic indices.

CONCLUSIONS

A fundamental step in the development of any effective attack on the general female population with the aim of early diagnosis is the identification of the woman at risk. Breast parenchymal patterns appear to offer the best method with the knowledge available today. Programs of surveillance could be developed based on all risk factors, but primarily on the radiographic one, so that we could space our early detection efforts at different intervals for different groups of patients. Although the hypothesis has not been tested, one could develop a reasonable screening study on the basis of the material studied thus far. For example, women in the N1 category starting at age 35 would be subject to stringent examination including mammography at perhaps five-year intervals before the age of 50. This would be contrasted to regimens for women classified as either P2 or DY for whom the recommendations would be for yearly mammographic studies until further knowledge can be gained to either shorten or lengthen the interval time; likely one would find that the interval could be lengthened slightly.

The correlative work between the radiologist and pathologist at this early stage is very encouraging and will be pursued further. In addition, further efforts at refinement of the radiographic risk patterns are currently underway and should be studied by others. Efforts should also be made to see if the radiographic risk patterns can be combined with other factors, such as patient's age, parity and family history to strengthen them.

REFERENCES

1. Wolfe, JN, Mammography: reports on its use in women with breasts abnormal and normal on physical examination. Radiology 83:244-254, 1964

2. Wolfe, JN, A study of breast parenchyma by mammography in the normal woman and those with benign and malignant disease. Radiology 89:201-205, 1967

3. Wolfe, JN, Risk for breast cancer development determined by mammographic parenchymal pattern. Cancer 37:2486-2492, 1976

4. Wolfe, JN, Breast patterns as an index of risk for developing breast cancer. Am J Roentgenol 126:1130-1139, 1976

5. Mendell, L, M Rosenbloom and A Naimark, Are breast patterns a risk index of breast cancer? A reappraisal. Am J Roentgenol 128:547, 1977

6. Egan, RL and RC Mosteller, Breast cancer mammography patterns. Cancer 40(5):2087-2090, 1977

7. Krook, PM, T Carlile, W Bush, et al, Mammographic parenchymal patterns as a risk indicator for prevalent and incident cancer. Cancer 41:1093-1097, 1978

8. Wilkinson, E, C Clopton, J Gordonson, et al, Mammography parenchymal pattern and the risk of breast cancer. Natl Cancer Inst 59:1397-1400, 1977

9. Hainline, S, L Myers, R McLelland, et al, Mammographic patterns and risk of breast cancer. Am J Roentgenol 130:1157-1158, 1978

10. Wolfe, MD, Breast parenchymal patterns: prevalent and incident carcinomas. Radiology 131:267-268, 1979

11. Wellings, SR, and JN Wolfe, Correlative studies of the histological and radiographic appearance of breast parenchyma. Radiology 129:299-306, 1978

12. Wellings, SR, HM Jensen and RG Marcus, An atlas of subgross pathology of the human breast with special reference to possible precancerous lesions. J Natl Cancer Inst 55:231-273, 1975

13. Wellings, SR and HM Jensen, On the origin and progression of ductal carcinoma in the human breast. J Natl Cancer Inst 50:1111-1118, 1973

14. Jensen, HM, JR Rice and SR Wellings, Preneoplastic lesions in the human breast. Science 191:295-297, 1976

15. Black, MM, THC Barclay, SJ Cutler, et al, Association of atypical characteristics of benign breast lesions with subsequent risk of breast cancer. Cancer 29:338-343, 1972

INITIAL MANAGEMENT OF CARCINOMA OF THE BREAST WITH RADIATION THERAPY INSTEAD OF MASTECTOMY

Leonard R. Prosnitz, M.D.

Yale University School of Medicine

New Haven, Connecticut

INTRODUCTION

Cancer of the breast remains the most common form of cancer in women in the United States, with an estimated 100,000 new cases and 34,000 deaths in 1979. It is also undoubtedly the most controversial malignancy in terms of its management. Historically, attempts to improve the cure rate of this disease have focused on different approaches to local therapy, such as performing a more extensive operation or adding radiation to inaccessible lymph nodes. These attempts have been based on the notion that breast cancer begins as a single focus and spreads in an orderly fashion to regional lymph nodes before it disseminates to distant sites.

A large body of evidence, however, recently reviewed by Fisher (1), is accumulating to refute this concept. It is probable that breast cancer is often disseminated at the time of presentation; that positive axillary nodes, for example, are a harbinger of dissemination rather than a localized extension of cancer which must be eliminated to cure the patient. Data from the National Surgical Adjuvant Breast Project (NSABP) and from our own institution indicate that 60-80% of patients with 4 or more axillary nodes involved with cancer will have relapsed by 5 years (2,3). Attention has therefore shifted to some extent to the problem of dealing with this dissemination with the use of "adjuvant" chemotherapy.

Further support for the Fisher thesis comes from a consideration of the vast numbers of published papers on alternate methods of primary management of breast cancer. Despite the enthusiasm many authors have for their particular treatment, survival appears to be about the same no matter what the local treatment.

Even if survival differences are minimal, the local management of primary breast cancer is not a trivial issue - ask any woman who has had a breast removed. If different types of local therapy do not substantially alter the breast cancer cure rate, it behooves the clinician to use that type of local treatment that will be associated with the least morbidity and produce the best cosmetic, functional, and psychological result. If amputation of the breast can be avoided by the use of radiation, this is likely to be of great psychological benefit to the patient.

Data are now accumulating from our own institution, as well as a number of other centers, that radiation therapy to the intact breast and draining lymph nodes combined with surgical removal of the mass ("lumpectomy", excisional biopsy, partial mastectomy) results in a cure rate equivalent to more conventional procedures such as radical or modified radical mastectomy. In the hands of a skilled radiotherapist using proper equipment, the cosmetic results are excellent and the overall treatment morbidity minimal.

To understand fully the role of radiation therapy in the treatment of breast cancer, however, it is first necessary to review some basic radiobiological principles.

RADIOBIOLOGIC BASIS FOR THERAPY

Radiotherapy is recognized as an effective, curative treatment modality for many types of cancers, such as cancer of the head and neck or gynecologic malignancies such as cervical carcinoma. The ability of radiation to cure these tumors is obviously related to its ability to achieve local control. Doses necessary for local control are well established for head and neck cancer and cancer of the cervix. Generally, 6000-7000 rads (1000 rads per week, 5 fractions) is necessary to control small clinical masses (2-4 cm). Subclinical disease requires 4500-5000 rads (4).

Radiobiologic data obtained from tissue culture experiments indicate that the inherent radiosensitivity of most human tumors (both epidermoid and adenocarcinoma) is about the same (5). There is also a fairly large body of clinical data obtained from the radiation of advanced unresectable primary breast cancers, from the treatment of patients postoperatively following mastectomy and from the irradiation of local recurrences. Radiotherapeutic control is dependent both on the size of the tumor and the dose of radiation given with the dose response curve being of the usual sigmoid type. Clinically evident tumor requires a larger dose than subclinical disease. 3000-3500 rads (200 rads per fraction) will control 60-70% of subclinical disease, 4000 rads controls 80-85% and 4500-5000 rads results in local control in over 90% of cases (4). For small clinical masses (2-4 cm), doses of 6000-7000 rads in 6-7 weeks are necessary for 90% local control. For larger tumor masses, doses of up to 9000 rads may be required, and even so local control may not be achieved (6). Doses of 4000 rads or more can only be given safely with supervoltage equipment - with orthovoltage, complication rates are unacceptably high.

Large tumor masses are more resistant to radiation, probably because they contain significant numbers of hypoxic cells. Hypoxia does dramatically alter the inherent radiosensitivity of cancer cells, making them 2½-3 times less sensitive to radiation than well oxygenated tumors. In addition, the larger tumors may be more resistant to radiation simply because of the larger number of cells contained in them. These simple facts regarding the doses of radiation necessary for local control have often been ignored in the design of some of the more prominent and most widely quoted studies into the effects of radiation on breast cancer.

Historically, the role of radiotherapy in the management of locally advanced breast cancer and metastatic disease has been recognized for a long time. As well known a proponent of radical mastectomy as Haagensen stated in his textbook 20 years ago that patients with any one of five "grave" signs of disease should not have a mastectomy but have a better survival with radiotherapy alone (7). Later, Haagensen expanded the group of patients for whom he did not recommend radical mastectomy to include those women with clinically small disease but positive biopsies from either the apex of the axilla and/or the internal mammary lymph nodes. These patients were treated by Ruth Guttmann with radiation alone with a 30% 5-year survival in advanced disease (stage III) and a 50% 5-year survival in patients rejected for surgery because of positive node biopsies (8). This rather striking (relative) success of radiation in advanced disease leads to the question: Why not use radiation in early disease?

Despite the controversy over the effects of postoperative (i.e. post-mastectomy) irradiation on survival of the patient, there is little doubt that local recurrence is markedly diminished when radiotherapy is added to surgery. Again, one must raise the question: If radiotherapy can successfully control disease in lymph nodes and on the chest wall, why not rely on it to do the same in the breast itself? It is very instructive to read virtually the same argument advanced by McWhirter 25 years ago (9).

On theoretic grounds then, radiation should be able to easily kill small numbers of cancer cells within the breast after the main tumor mass has been excised. Removal of the lump itself reduces the chance of hypoxic cells being present and also reduces the dose of radiation necessary for local control with less likelihood of adverse effects on normal tissue.

PRINCIPLES OF PRIMARY RADIATION THERAPY

The above biologic information suggests that primary radiotherapy should be equally effective as surgery for achieving local control of breast cancer, provided one adheres to a few basic principles. These are as follows:

(1) The gross tumor mass should be excised, reducing the dose of radiation necessary and in turn leading to a better cosmetic result. Wide local excision is not necessary; just the lump itself needs to be removed. If the mass is large relative to the size of the breast itself, then mastectomy may be necessary in order to comfortably remove the mass, or the cosmetic defect may be large enough so that preservation of the remaining breast is not worthwhile.

(2) The radiation dose needs to be about 5000 rads to all areas at risk for subclinical disease. We usually boost the area of the tumor itself with an additional 1000-1500 rads (either with external beam treatment or by means of a radioactive implant). Strictly speaking, this boost dose may not be necessary but can easily be done without adding significantly to morbidity.

(3) The area irradiated should be the entire breast, supraclavicular, axillary and internal mammary lymph nodes, the radiation equivalent of an extended radical mastectomy. It is by no means certain that this large a radiation field is necessary, but this kind of treatment can be done with minimal morbidity and is conceivably beneficial in terms of survival, although by no means proven.

(4) Supervoltage equipment, careful treatment planning with the use of wedged fields in order to achieve a uniform dose distribution, careful matching of adjacent fields to avoid overlap, and avoidance of bolus are all important technical details to which attention must be paid if one is to get a good cosmetic result. It must be kept in mind that improvement in appearance and a better psychological and functional end result is the chief reason for using radiation instead of surgery and that particular attention must be paid to radiation technique in order to minimize morbidity. Otherwise, surgery might just as well be performed.

(5) Obese women and/or those with large, pendulous breasts are often not suitable for primary radiotherapy, as it is quite difficult to achieve uniform dose distribution or reproduce the treatment field precisely from day to day. In addition, larger quantities of fat within the breast tend to result in a greater amount of fibrosis in the years following treatment. Accordingly, we do not consider such patients to be suitable candidates for primary radiation and often recommend mastectomy.

RESULTS OF PRIMARY RADIOTHERAPY

The most important question, of course, is whether patients treated with radiation as primary management of their breast cancer instead of mastectomy have, in fact, a survival equivalent to those treated with more conventional surgical procedures. We believe sufficient data have now accumulated in the United States, Europe and Canada to answer this question. One of the earliest reports of the efficacy of radiotherapy without mastectomy as primary management of breast cancer appeared in 1954 from Helsinki. Mustakalloi described a 5-year survival of 84% in 127 stage I patients treated with excision plus radiation (10). A followup report from the same instutution in 1969 by Rissanen described a 5-year survival of 79% in 415 stage I and II patients (11).

At the Princess Margaret Hospital in Toronto, Vera Peters reported a matched pair analysis of 300 stage I patients, half of whom received local excision and irradiation and the other half mastectomy and postoperative irradiation, all of whom were followed for a period of 5-35 years. Sixty-seven per cent of the irradiated group were free of disease compared with 58% of the mastectomy group, not a significant difference but certainly no worse in the irradiated patients (12).

Spitalier (Marseilles, France) described 276 stage I and II patients treated with irradiation (with or without local excision) (13). The disease-free survival was 85% at 5 years in stage I patients and 71% in stage II patients. In patients in whom local excision had been done, these numbers increased to 90% and 79% respectively. Spitalier also made the very interesting observation that of those patients who did develop a local recurrence and subsequently had to undergo a mastectomy, half were alive and free of disease at 5 years following mastectomy, so that local recurrence after irradiation as primary treatment does not carry the same ominous prognosis that is usually associated with local recurrence following mastectomy.

One negative report on primary radiotherapy that is often quoted is the Guy's Hospital randomized trial that compared excision plus radiation with radical mastectomy and postoperative irradiation (14). In stage I patients, the survival for both treatment groups was the same at 10 years, although local recurrence in the excision plus radiation group was about 20%. In stage II patients, however, the mastectomy group has a 55% survival vs 25% for the excision group (p .05). It is not generally appreciated, however, that the radiation doses used in this trial were totally inadequate by current standards. The breast received 3500-3800 rads and the lymph nodes 2500-2700 rads.

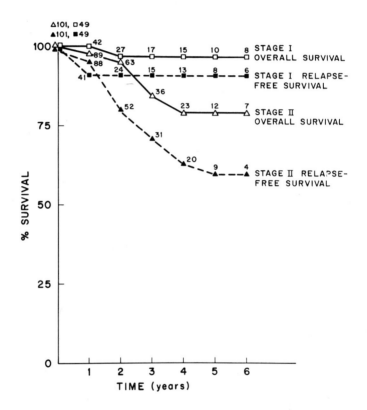

Figure 1: Cumulative overall survival and relapse-free survival of Stage I and II patients treated with radiation.

Table 1

Author	Clinical Stage	No. of Pts.	Type of Mastectomy*	Postop Radiotherapy	5-Year Survival (%)	Age Corrected	Local Recurrence Rate (%)
Brinkley	I	159	R,MR, Total	Yes	83	Yes	
	II	119	Total	Yes	58	Yes	
	II	93	R	Yes	52	Yes	
Butcher	A	216	R	+Nodes	76	No	
	B	135	R	+Nodes	48	No	
Dahl-Iversen	A	312	ER	No	78	No	20
	B	67	ER	No	46	No	32
Fisher	I & II	414	R	No	63	No	11
Haagensen	A	344	R	5%	85	No	7
	B	138	R	12%	59	No	18
Handley	A	77	MR	+Nodes	75	No	16
	B	58	MR	+Nodes	57	No	26
Kaae	A	157	Total	Yes	70	No	19
	B	28	Total	Yes	50	No	29
Urban	I	236	ER	+Nodes	81	No	2
Williams	A	68	MR	Yes	72	No	22
	B	57	MR	Yes	60	No	26

*R = Radical, ER = Extended Radical, MR = Modified Radical

In the United States, radiotherapy without mastectomy has remained a distinctly uncommon procedure. Our own interest goes back 10 to 12 years, but in the early years most patients being treated were referred because they were considered to be inoperable. Gradually, however, some surgeons have begun to refer patients for this procedure for other than medical contraindications to surgery. Most of our patients, however, are self-referred - they have chosen to carefully explore all options of treatment available rather than quickly submitting to mastectomy.

Nevertheless, the numbers of patients treated with radiotherapy alone at any one U.S. institution remain quite small. We therefore decided to combine data from four institutions with a similar interest and philosophy of treatment - Harvard, Yale, Jefferson Medical College, and Hahnemann in Philadelphia. One hundred patients with clinical stage I and II breast cancer (UICC-AJC) treated at these four centers with local excision and radiation were reported in Cancer in 1977 (15). Approximately 250 have now been treated.

Treatment results are shown in figure 1. In stage I patients, the overall 5-year survival is 97%, the relapse-free survival 92%. Clinical stage II patients have an 80% 5-year survival overall, and a 60% relapse-free 5-year survival. None of these patients has had an axillary lymph node dissection or received adjuvant chemotherapy.

At the M.D. Anderson Hospital in Houston, 82 stage I and II patients receiving primary radiotherapy without mastectomy had a 5-year relapse-free survival of 80% and an overall survival of 90% (16).

It is interesting that the 5-year disease-free rates in clinical stage I patients are so high when we know that 30% of clinical stage I patients have axillary nodal involvement microscopically (17). The explanation appears to be that in patients who are thought clinically to be stage I, the surgical discovery of positive axillary lymph nodes, particularly 3 or less, does not worsen the prognosis to the extent that it does in more advanced stages (3,7).

How do these results compare with more conventional treatment procedures such as radical or modified radical mastectomy, with or without postoperative radiotherapy? Such comparisons are very difficult to make for a variety of reasons: the non-random nature of case selection, different methods of staging, different ways of reporting results, e.g. relapse rates, overall survival, survival corrected for intercurrent disease, relapse-free survival, etc. Nevertheless, table 1 lists a number of the more prominent surgical series selected from the many available in the literature. Despite the heterogeniety of these studies, it is still apparent that 5-year survivals of 75-85% for stage I

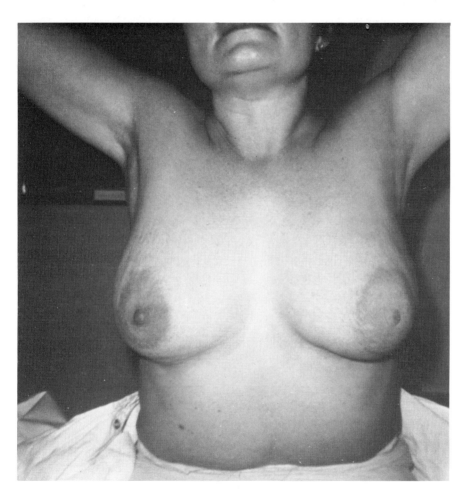

Figure 2: Appearance of a patient 4 years
after definitive radiotherapy to left breast.

patients are the rule and 50-60% for stage II patients, no matter what the treatment is. The few randomized prospective studies that are available from this country and elsewhere support the view that there is little difference among the treatment options. Randomized prospective studies to prove or disprove the merits of primary radiotherapy as opposed to mastectomy are not available as yet, although two such studies are in progress, one at the National Cancer Institute in Milan and the other an NSABP study. To date, these studies show no difference in any of the treatment groups. Although homage is always paid to the randomized prospective trial, we feel obligated to point out that modified radical mastectomy has probably replaced a radical mastectomy in most surgeons' minds as the procedure of choice, and there is not a single published randomized trial in the literature in support of this procedure.

Are the 5-year results too early to discuss or must one wait for the results at 10 years? Although there are many 5-year survivors who die between the 5th and 10th years, 85-90% of relapses occur before 5 years so that radiotherapy results that are reported in terms of relapse-free survival are very unlikely to change significantly with the passage of time.

Local recurrences, i.e. relapse of breast cancer within the irradiated field, either in the breast or nodes, took place in 10 patients (all in the breast) of our series of 150 patients, an incidence of 6.6%. Similar to the Spitalier series mentioned above, 5 of these 10 patients are disease free for prolonged periods after mastectomy. This incidence of local recurrence is virtually the same as that observed following radical mastectomy and postoperative irradiation in stage I and II patients.

The cosmetic results obtained have generally been excellent (figure 2). With suitable patients (i.e. not too obese) and with attention to technical detail as mentioned earlier, almost all patients will have only a minimum of radiation changes. We cannot overemphasize the emotional benefits that patients derive by avoiding mastectomy, at no compromise to their ultimate survival.

COMPLICATIONS OF RADIOTHERAPY

Complications from primary radiotherapy of breast cancer are, fortunately, few. During the acute phase of treatment problems are generally minimal, consisting of fatigue, very infrequent nausea, and a brisk erythema over the treated area towards the completion of therapy. Problems developing during the weeks and months following radiation are of much more importance. Potentially, the most troublesome of these is radiation pneumonitis which may occur with a frequency of 1-10% (18). Chest X-ray changes are considerably more common than clinical symptoms. In our 150 patients, this complication was seen in 4, all of whom recovered spontaneously without the use of corticosteroids. The frequency of radiation pneumonitis can be kept to a minimum by careful attention to the amount of underlying lung included in the tangential port films.

Some degree of fibrosis in the treated breast with slight shrinkage and retraction is usually seen. Thickened nodules may develop along matchlines between the treated fields which are usually not disturbing to the patient but may be confused by the unwary with recurrent breast cancer.

Other complications observed in our series included rib fractures, arm edema and pleural effusion. The total incidence of these problems was 3%, and at least some of them were related to an unusual fractionation scheme that was employed at one time by one of the institutions.

Other potential problems from radiation include impaired immunity and increase in secondary malignancies. The evidence concerning immune alterations is complex and contradictory. Certainly the clinical results do not suggest any adverse effect of radiation on immune responses at least as reflected in survival. Radiation-induced breast cancers from low doses of radiation such as those used in mammography have been reported, and some increased frequency of this would be anticipated (19). It is also known, however, that the frequency of radiation-induced cancer tends to decrease above a certain dose of radiation in the therapeutic range (20). A radiation-induced malignancy in the treated breast would not be distinguishable from a local recurrence, and since the overall frequency of local recurrence in our series and in most series is approximately 5%, well below that of most surgical series, it is doubtful that radiation-induced malignancies will be a problem of any magnitude.

RELATIONSHIP OF PRIMARY RADIATION TO ADJUVANT CHEMOTHERAPY

One of the arguments often advanced for surgical therapy is that it is necessary to do a radical or modified radical mastectomy in order to look at axillary lymph nodes to select patients for adjuvant chemotherapy or otherwise determine prognosis. This argument is without foundation, since if one wants to sample axillary lymph nodes or do a full axillary dissection, this has nothing to do with the performance of a mastectomy, and the breast could still be left in place for treatment with radiation. In fact, we recommend axillary dissection in women with palpable axillary lymph nodes, since administration of more than 5000 rads to the axilla is likely to result in excessive morbidity. We also recommend an axillary sampling procedure for premenopausal women in order to select patients for adjuvant chemotherapy.

Radiation therapy may compromise the ability to administer subsequent adjuvant chemotherapy because of interference with hematologic tolerance. In addition, the normal tissue reactions caused by approximately 5000 rads to large fields may be enhanced by the subsequent administration of chemotherapy. For example, in the author's personal series at Yale, no rib fractures had been encountered in primarily irradiated patients until the use of adjuvant chemo-therapy; however, subsequent to that time several patients receiving both modalities have had this complication. Evidence on all these points is largely anecdotal at the present time, but the two randomized trials of primary radiotherapy currently in progress both employ chemotherapy as well so that these answers should be forthcoming.

CONCLUSIONS

Considerable evidence has been marshalled to show that local excision combined with radiation therapy is as effective as mastectomy in the primary management of breast cancer. Admittedly, the experience with this procedure is not nearly as extensive as that with more conventional surgical procedures. We have entered an era, however, of much more extensive participation by the patient in decisions concerning her medical care. We hope that those who remain dubious as to the wisdom of primary radiotherapy will at least inform that patient that this option exists and enable her to participate more directly in the decision making process. Let the patient see a radiotherapist in consultation prior to mastectomy and have the therapeutic options explained to her by both surgeon and radiotherapist. Perhaps as women become aware that there are other options besides mastectomy for the treatment of breast cancer, that the diagnosis does not automatically mean loss of the breast, they may seek medical attention sooner with smaller lesions and thus a real improvement in cure rates may result.

REFERENCES

1. Fisher, B, Biological and clinical considerations regarding the use of surgery and chemotherapy in the treatment of primary breast cancer. Cancer 40:574-587, 1977

2. Fisher, B, NH Slack, DL Katrych, N Wolmark, Ten year follow-up of results of patients with carcinoma of the breast in a cooperative clinical trial evaluating surgical adjuvant chemotherapy. Surg Gyencol Obstet 140:528-534, 1975

3. Packard, RA, LR Prosnitz, SN Bobrow, Selection of breast cancer patients for adjuvant chemotherapy: another look at the prognostic significance of involved lymph nodes. JAMA 238:1034-1036, 1977

4. Fletcher, GH, Clinical dose-response curves of human malignant epithelial tumors. Brit J Radiol 46:1-12, 1973

5. Andrews, JR, The Radiobiology of Human Cancer Radiotherapy. Philadelphia, W.B.Saunders, 1968

6. Fletcher, GH, Local results of irradiation in the primary management of localized breast cancer. Cancer 29:545-551, 1972

7. Haagensen, CD, Diseases of the Breast. 1st ed. Philadelphia, W.B. Saunders, 1956

8. Guttmann, R, Radiotherapy in locally advanced cancer of the breast. Cancer 20:1046-1050, 1967

9. McWhirter, R, Simple mastectomy and radiotherapy in the treatment of breast cancer. Brit J Radiol 28:128-139, 1955

10. Mustakallio, S, Treatment of breast cancer by tumor extirpation and roentgen therapy instead of radical operation. J Fac Radiol 6:23-26, 1954

11. Rissanen, PM, A comparison of conservative and radical surgery combined with radiotherapy in the treatment of stage I carcinoma of the breast. Brit J Radiol 42:423-426, 1969

12. Peters, MV, Cutting the "Gordian Knot" in early breast cancer. Ann Royal Coll Phys Surg Can 8:186-192, 1975

13. Spitalier, J, H Brandon, Y Ayme, et al, Cesium therapy of breast cancer: a 5-year report on 400 consecutive patients. Int J Rad Oncol 2:231-235, 1977

14. Atkins, H, JL Hayward, DJ Klugman, AB Wayte, Treatment of early breast cancer - a report after 10 years of a clinical trial. Brit Med J 2:423-429, 1972

196

15. Prosnitz, LR, IS Goldenberg, RA Packard, et al, Radiation therapy as initial treatment for early¯ stage cancer of the breast without mastectomy. Cancer 39:917-923, 1977

16. Fletcher, GH, E Montague, AJ Nelson, Combination of conservative surgery and irradiation for cancer of the breast. Amer J Roent 126:216-222, 1976

17. Cutler, SJ, LM Axtel, D Schottenfeld, et al, Clinical assessment of lymph nodes in carcinoma of the breast. Surg Gynec Obstet 131:41-52, 1970

18. Fletcher, GH, Textbook of Radiotherapy. 2nd ed. Philadelphia, Lea and Febiger, 1973

19. National Research Council Advisory Committee on the Biological Effects of Ionizing Radiation: The effects on populations of exposure to low levels of ionizing radiation: Report. Washington, D.C., National Academy of Sciences - National Research Council, 1972

20. Hutchinson, GB, Late neoplastic changes following medical irradiation. Cancer 37:1102-1107, 1976

THE SURGICAL TREATMENT OF PRIMARY BREAST CANCER

Richard G. Margolese

Centre Hospitalier

Jewish General Hospital

Montreal, Canada

THE RADICAL MASTECTOMY

The surgical approach to the treatment of primary breast cancer has remained unchanged and virtually unchallenged for the better part of 8 decades. During this time, there has developed an almost biblical reverence for the Halstead radical mastectomy; this allegiance now deserves a belated review and perhaps revision.

Historical Perspective

A review of Halstead's original publication indicates that he formed his ideas about surgical treatment based on the then existing concepts of anatomy and lymphatic physiology. Together with W.S.Handley, Halstead had developed the idea that cancer spread by direct lymphatic permeation. It was this erroneous view which led to the evolution of the Radical Mastectomy to treat breast cancer (1). This approach even considered amputation of the humerus for bony metastases and amputation of the hip for femoral head involvement as part of the "en bloc" approach. Halstead further postulated that the liver became involved by direct contiguous permeation via the linea alba and round ligament (1). These ideas were the natural product of the existing concept of lymphatic routes of cancer spread.

The resulting procedure, the Radical Mastectomy, has never been properly compared as a reference operation to other operations and few of today's surgeons have stopped to re-evaluate this operation from a modern point of view. It is often said that this operation has "stood the test of time". In truth there has been no real test and surgeons continue to adhere to the Radical or the Modified Radical Mastectomy, more out of a sense of tradition than scientific merit or justification. In fact, when measured against a group of contemporary cases not treated by Radical Mastectomy, it appears that the Halstead operation had very little impact on long term survival.

Although there was a dramatic reduction of the local recurrence rate due to the radical mastectomy, the 10-year survival for Halstead's patients was only 12%. The comparative figure at that time was 9%. This small increase in survival can best be attributed to a reduction in operative mortality which was due, in turn, to other innovations of Halstead but not necessarily to the "en bloc" operation itself. The failure of the introduction of Radical Mastectomy to improve real survival figures is most easily explained by analysis of the type of cases seen. The society of Halstead's times was basically rural; urban hospitals and concepts of early diagnosis, as we know them, did not exist. It is probable that Halstead saw what we now consider to be inoperable cases with large tumors, perhaps displaying skin retraction or fixation, satellite lesions, and other so called grave signs. Although for local control, the Radical Mastectomy was more effective than simple excision, cure in these cases was not obtainable. In later decades, more suitable earlier cases gave better results, and surgeons never asked if the operation was truly the cause for this improvement.

Current Perspective

Since it is now clear that Halstead's preliminary concepts were in error, we should examine the validity of the Halstead Radical Mastectomy as a curative operation. This question has been approached by several investigators over the past 2 decades and some comparative trials have been conducted (2-6). In the main, they show that there is apparent equivalence between radical mastectomy, radical mastectomy with regional lymph node radiation, extended radical mastectomy, and simple mastectomy alone, although these conclusions are less often accepted than challenged, or ignored, by most surgeons.

TREATMENT OF AXILLARY NODES

Much of the debate about appropriate surgery has centered on the role of axillary lymph nodes, and two opposing views predominate. On the one hand is the radical approach which suggests that 70% of palpable nodes contain tumor on pathological exam; 30% of nodes which are not palpable may still contain tumor. Since positive nodes may be a source of spread with lethal outcome they should be removed as expeditiously and completely as possible. On the other hand, the conservative approach conceives of palpable nodes as having reactive hyperplasia in 30% of cases, and non-palpable nodes as being truly negative in perhaps 70% of cases. Since positive nodes are a sign of systemic, incurable disease, excision is futile and removal of some types of palpable nodes might even be detrimental. Therefore, there is no justification for treating the axillary lymph nodes.

Unfortunately, this debate was not resolved by any of the above studies. Many of the studies were retrospective or had design flaws which caused observers to be critical of the findings. It can be said that the vast majority of practicing surgeons did not abandon the Radical Mastectomy as a result of these studies. In order to provide an answer to the problem of lymph node treatment in Radical Mastectomy the National Surgical Adjuvant Breast Project launched a study in 1971 comparing Radical Mastectomy versus Total Mastectomy with regional lymph node radiation, versus Total Mastectomy alone, i.e., no treatment to axillary lymph nodes at all (figure 1).

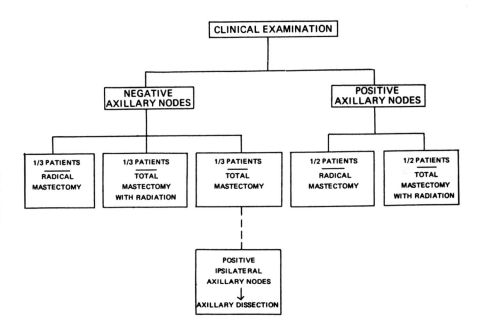

Figure 1: Schema for NSABP Protocol #4 comparing Radical Mastectomy and Total Mastectomy with or without postoperative radiation therapy.

These treatments were applied to 980 patients with clinically negative axillary lymph nodes. A further group of 501 patients with clinically positive lymph nodes were treated by Radical Mastectomy or total mastectomy with nodal radiation but were not subjected to a third treatment arm. The National Surgical Adjuvant Breast Project has reported that at 60 months there is no significant difference between the treatments evaluated (7,8). That is, patients with positive nodes had equal treatment failure rates and equal survival rates whether they were treated by Radical Mastectomy or Total Mastectomy and radiation. Similarly, patients with negative nodes have equal failure and survival rates with any of the three treatment arms (figure 2).

200

LIFE TABLE PROBABILITY(%) OF <u>SURVIVAL</u> BY MONTHS AFTER MASTECTOMY

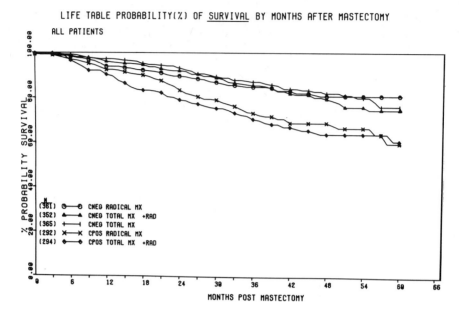

Figure 2: Results of NSABP Protocol #4

This prospective, randomized, controlled clinical trial involving 1,481 patients constitutes strong evidence that treatment of the axillary lymph nodes by surgery, radiotherapy or no treatment at all, does not influence survival in breast cancer. This is turn implies that local management of the lymph nodes is not a factor in determining ultimate prognosis for patients with breast cancer. In fact, most evidence indicates that lymph nodes involved with tumor are not a source of distant metastases but merely a sign that metastases have occurred. Spratt (9) has shown that the time from surgery to appearance of local recurrence is the same as the time from surgery to distant recurrences, further proof that local recurrence is not the precursor of widespread disease. The old concept that cancer spreads from a primary site to regional lymph nodes and from there in time, to distant sites is, therefore, no longer valid. The modern view is that cancer cells are circulating very early in that cancer's development, and other factors are responsible for the ability of these cells to settle in a capillary bed, remain viable and grow as metastases.   Fisher (10) has demonstrated the existence of veno-lymphatic interconnections and it is likely that metastases are simultaneously hematogenous and lymphatic in origin.

PREDICTIVE VALUE OF AXILLARY LYMPH NODES

The most disturbing point of these various studies on lymph node status is the realization that breast cancer is not very curable. A review of a previous National Surgical Adjuvant Breast Project study showed the astonishing predictive power that lymph node status has on eventual outcome. In a group of Radical Mastectomy patients in this study, 73% of those with negative nodes were free from recurrence at the 10-year interval, but over 86% of patients with 4 or more positive nodes had experienced treatment failure by that date. The failure rate for patients with 1-3 positive nodes was 65% (11). Thus, the vast majority of patients with pathologically involved lymph nodes will not survive, regardless of the extent of surgery.

It is particularly distressing to note that these figures were obtained in a group of cases who presented with clinical Stage I and Stage II disease, who were therefore considered potentially curable and were subjected to radical mastectomy as a curative operation. It is obvious that these patients were not helped by this major surgery which has devastating cosmetic results.

If surgical or radiotherapeutic treatment of axillary lymph nodes does not prevent distant metastases it must be because those patients who ultimately fail already have their metastases established at the time these treatments are instituted. This concept has profound implications for choosing appropriate surgical treatment. Planning more radical operations to obtain cure is therefore not pertinent to the real problem.

LESSER SURGICAL PROCEDURES

Rationale

Although we do not have the means to identify prospectively all those patients who do have good prognoses, clearly, there is a group of patients who will do well with any surgery. Frequently, these patients have no residual tumor after biopsy. This group usually includes those with small tumors and good host-defense characteristics. Conversely, there is a group of patients for whom no operation will be curative. This group is made up of all those patients who eventually will fail following radical surgery. They often have larger tumors, clinically positive nodes, and may display other grave signs. However, the majority of these apparently predetermined cases are indistinguishable from patients for whom the extent of surgery might make a difference, if indeed such a group exists (figure 3).

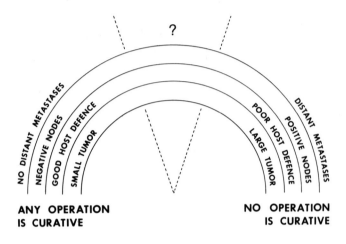

Figure 3

It is not known whether such a middle group does, in fact, exist. There is mounting evidence that local control of the tumor is only one aspect of proper treatment and perhaps this can often be obtained with lesser operations. More extensive local or regional surgery is not necessary and does not help because the problem is not local or regional.

Results of Prior Trials

This leads to the next consideration in primary breast cancer surgery: that of segmental mastectomy which also goes under the name of tylectomy, lumpectomy or partial mastectomy. There are several reports in the last 15 to 20 years indicating that his operation compares favorably with the classical Radical and Modified Radical Mastectomy. Foremost among these is Mustakalio in Finland who reported 10 and 20 year follow-up on 702 patients with the same survival rates for a Radical Mastectomy group (12,13). Peters' report of a 10-year retrospective match showed equivalent recurrence and survival rates for a

Radical Mastectomy group and an excisional biospy and radiation group (14). Other contributions by Wise (15), Adair (16), Porrit (17), and Crile (18) report the same conclusions (table 1).

Table 1

SEGMENTAL MASTECTOMY

MUSTAKALIO	702 pts.	Consecutive cases 10, 20 years
PETERS	434 pts.	Retrospective match. 10 years
WISE	186 pts.	Retrospective match. 10 years
ADAIR	24 pts.	1943 no match
PORRIT	183 pts.	Selected cases 5 years
CRILE	465 pts.	Retrospective match. 15 years
ATKINS	370 cases	Prospective controls. 10 years

The only prospective trial was led by Atkins (19) in the United Kingdom and involved 370 cases, comparing excisional biopsy plus axillary radiation versus radical mastectomy. For clinical Stage I patients, the 5 and 10 year survival rates were identical for the two treatment groups. However, in Stage II patients, only the 5 year survival rates were equivalent. At 10 years the radical mastectomy group did better than the local resections and radiation group. Closer analysis, however, is necessary before reaching a conclusion about this study. A review of sites of recurrence in this study indicates that, contrary to what many expected, local breast and chest wall recurrence was not a major factor in treatment failure. Axillary recurrence, however, was seen in 22% of patients in the excision and radiation group and in only 1% of the radical mastectomy group. This is unusually high and requires further explanation.

On analysis, it is apparent that the difference in survival was related mainly to axillary recurrence. It should be noted that the axillary radiation used was 2700 rads. This is well below what is now viewed as a tumoricidal dose and may very well have played a role in altering tumor antigenicity or host defenses so as to favor the growth of axillary metastases, producing a higher failure rate than might have been obtained had radiation not been given. There is experimental evidence to support this hypothesis. Schabel (20) has shown that in many different animal models, aliquots of transplanted tumor cells can be rendered more lethal by partial irradiation. In other words, fewer irradiated cells are necessary to produce lethal outcome than similar non-irradiated cells when injected into a variety of experimental animals.

Since most Stage I patients had negative axillary nodes this factor was not important in determining outcome. But the Stage II patients with positive nodes may have had a detrimental dose of radiation to involved nodes, reducing survival in the patients radiated, and causing the excision and radiation group to perform worse than the radical mastectomy group who had these nodes excised. This explanation is further reinforced by the National Surgical Adjuvant Breast Project findings that Radical Mastectomy, or Total Mastectomy and adequate axillary irradiation, gave the same results as not treating the axillary nodes (7). In addition, the McWhirter trial (2) and the Kings Hospital trial (21) also indicated that simple mastectomy and adequate irradiation or no irradiation were equal to radical mastectomy alone. Thus the use of partial irradiation has obscured the overall results in the Atkins trial. Because of this fault in design, the question of local excision cannot be answered in the context of this particular study, but there is sufficient evidence to justify another study with a more appropriate design. The National Surgical Adjuvant Breast Project has introduced such a trial which is now underway. This trial uses irradiation of the breast, but not of the lymph nodes, in one of its treatment arms. This radiation is introduced to deal with a fundamental biological aspect of breast cancer - that of multicentric, occult breast cancer, which may be a factor influencing the chance for local control by limited surgery.

MULTICENTRIC BREAST CANCER

Anatomical multicentricity

The true incidence of multicentric breast cancer is not clear. Mastectomy specimens, analyzed by stepwise section, have shown an incidence varying from 13-35% of patients, a range which clearly depends on the pathologist's interpretation of minimal breast cancer or atypical hyperplasia (22-25). Many of these foci are non-invasive and can be viewed as precancerous lesions or carcinoma-in-situ depending on terminology. Much controversy rages about the importance of these lesions and traditionalists who favor radical mastectomy claim that these foci could be a source of recurrent or second cancers and would ultimately cause treatment failure in a breast treated by a limited operation. The anatomical incidence, however, is not the true dimension of the problem and does not correlate with what appears to be the biologic importance, or lack of importance of these foci. In Crile's follow-up of 601 patient-years of exposure after partial mastectomy, six new cancers appeared in the contralateral breast and four in the affected one (23). Thus the danger for recurrence in the affected breast is less than might have been anticipated. Moreover, the breast is demonstrated to be a bilateral organ and consideration of multicentricity must include both breasts. The bilateral indicence of breast cancer, determined by random biopsies of the contralateral breast is reported by Urban (26) to be 14%, and by Sandison (23) to be 25%. If these lesions are important, the clinical incidence of contralateral breast cancer should be as high.

Clinical Multicentricity

However, Slack, Nemoto and Fisher (27) reviewed 2,734 cases and found the overall clinical incidence of a second contralateral primary breast cancer to be only 1.9% in a 6-year follow-up period. The majority of these were in patients with large primary tumors and in patients with positive axillary lymph nodes. These authors computed the possible advantages of performing a contralateral mastectomy on all patients with breast cancer and estimated that 5-year survival would increase by 0.8%.

Another approach to this problem is to look at a series of cases with lobular carcinoma-in-situ treated by biopsy only, and determine the true incidence of eventual cancer. McDivitt et al. (28) found an ultimate cancer rate of 25% in patients with lobular carcinoma-in-situ and concluded that Total Mastectomy was appropriate. Haagenson (29) reported an incidence of 22% but felt, however, that Total Mastectomy was inappropriate and that excisional biopsy and observation was the treatment of choice. Wheeler (30) reviewed a more extensive series of cases and found an incidence of 4%. Furthermore, he claimed that his figures were on much firmer statistical ground than the McDivitt or Haagenson figures, due mainly to his 100% follow-up at 20 years. In fact, the 95% confidence limits for the McDivitt study are so wide that they overlapped Wheeler's much narrower limits (figure 4).

The most interesting finding in these retrospective studies, however, is the revelation that in a collected group of 22 invasive cancers which did develop in patients who previously had lobular carcinoma-in-situ, 11 were in the ipsilateral breast, 8 in the contralateral breast, and 3 were bilateral (31). Moreover, only 6 of the 22 were small cell carcinoma, 10 were infiltrating ductal, and the remainder were tubular, medullary, or intraductal. This indicates that although there may be an increased risk for invasive cancer in these patients, a specific site of carcinoma-in-situ may not be the same site at which the subsequent cancer develops. If surgical therapy is based on the possibility that multi-focal disease exists, then unilateral mastectomy is only a half measure. A radical mastectomy would, therefore, have to be bilateral or it loses its logic.

INVESTIGATIVE SURGICAL APPROACH

Clearly, there is a valid controversy about the importance of multi-focal neoplasia and, obviously, the solution will not be obtained by anatomical and pathological debate. The prospective clinical trial being conducted by the National Surgical Adjuvant Breast Project is designed to answer this question. This compares segmental resection or segmental resection plus breast radiation versus total mastectomy. All 3 arms undergo axillary node dissection for staging purposes and all patients with positive nodes receive a standard 2-drug adjuvant chemotherapy. Negative node patients are not given further treatment (table 2).

Table 2

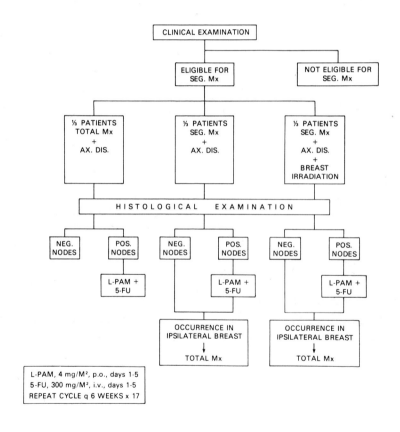

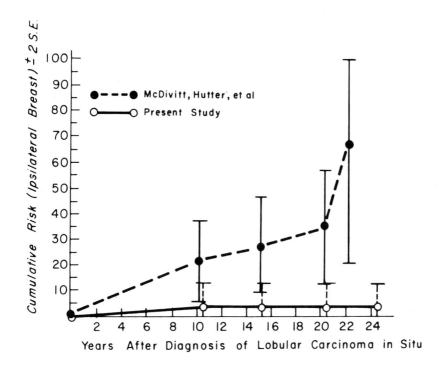

Figure 4: Wheeler: Incidence of Invasive carcinoma following Ca-in-situ (30).

Thus the only variables are the extent of surgery and the addition of radiotherapy to half of the patients undergoing segmental resection. This will indicate whether segmental resection alone is equally curative when compared with total mastectomy. The addition of radiotherapy to one half of the segmental patients will indicate whether multi-focal disease is important in terms of long term control, and, if it is, whether or not radiation therapy will manage it successfully.

It is hoped that this study will confirm the adequacy of limited surgery. If so, this will benefit many patients who now undergo breast amputation unnecessarily; however, it will not, by itself, improve overall cure rates. In fact, breast cancer death rates have not changed in over 4 decades, despite the introduction of more extensive surgical practices. It is possible, however, that adjuvant chemotherapy, when added to adequate surgical procedures, may increase survival rates. It is important to realize that adjuvant chemotherapy is not being proposed as a mopping up method to secure control in cases where inadequate surgery is performed. A more proper perspective is that those cases of breast cancer who fail following surgery do so because metastases have occurred prior to the surgery. The adjuvant chemotherapy is administered in the hope of eliminating these occult metastases and producing cure. Segmental Mastectomy is proposed as an equivalent to total mastectomy in completely eradicating the local tumor. It is not viewed as a lesser procedure made safe by the advent of chemotherapy.

As can be seen in figure 5, the surgical specimen is not a simple excisional biopsy but represents a complete segmental resection of the tumor and an adequate axillary dissection. While conspicuously less than a traditional mastectomy, this is a scientifically conceived cancer operation designed to control the primary tumor by complete removal.

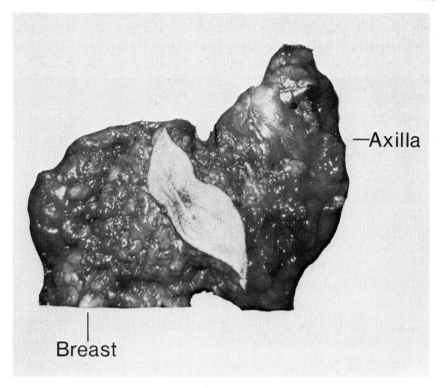

Figure 5: Surgical specimen from segmental resection.

Figure 6 shows the postoperative result, indicating that this approach is consistent with acceptable cosmetic results. Thus a modern view would shift from radical extensive "en bloc" resection for cure, to one of a less extensive surgical operation which is adequate for local control, combined with systemic treatment such as adjuvant chemotherapy which will, hopefully, achieve control of distant metastases if they exist. The National Surgical Adjuvant Breast Project Protocol #4 provided a test for the first part of this approach and the results support this view (7). As discussed above, treatment by Radical or total mastectomy, with or without radiotherapy produced no difference in failure rate. However, a clear difference in outome does exist for patients with positive axillary nodes compared to those with negative nodes even though all patients with nodes analyzed had the same treatment: Radical Mastectomy. Thus, while extent of surgery does not influence outcome, the presence of involved axillary nodes does (figure 7).

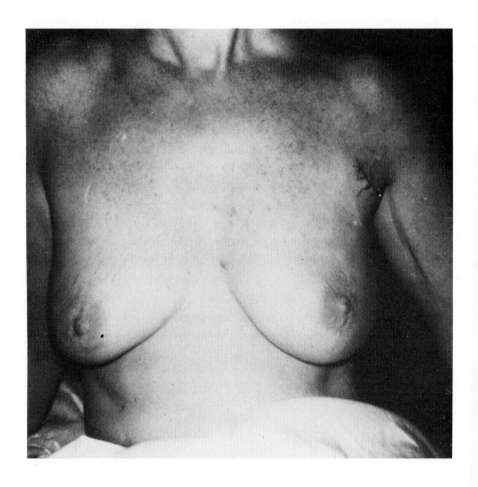

Figure 6: Postoperative results of segmental resection.

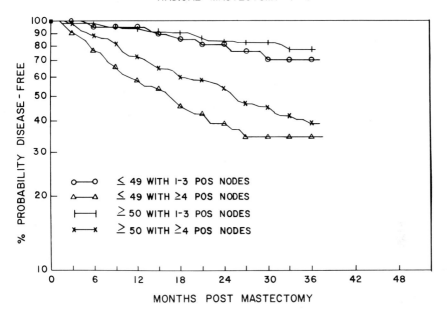

PROBABILITY (%) OF SURVIVAL WITHOUT DISEASE
RADICAL MASTECTOMY P-4

Figure 7

Axillary nodes, then, should be viewed as a marker for the presence of disseminated disease even if not yet clinically manifest. This identifies the group of patients who should be treated by adjuvant chemotherapy in the hope of eradicating these subclinical metastases.

ADJUVANT CHEMOTHERAPY

The concept of adjuvant chemotherapy, now 20 years old, began to undergo clinical trial soon after it was shown that cytotoxic drugs could induce remission in patients with disseminated breast cancer. Current approaches to adjuvant chemotherapy are based on animal models which have shown that tumors not cured by surgery alone or chemotherapy alone, can be cured when surgery and chemotherapy are combined (32).

The first clinical trial was based on the view, now seen as incorrect, that dissemination occurred at the time of surgery due to dislodgement of tumor cells by surgical manipulation. This was the National Surgical Adjuvant Breast Project trial (11) in which Thio-Tepa and 5-flourouracil were compared to placebo after radical mastectomy. The results indicated that Thio-Tepa provided a 20% improvement in 10-year survival rates for the subset of premenopausal women with 4 or more lymph nodes involved. With further understanding of tumor growth and kinetics, it was realized that pre-existing occult micrometastases and not surgical dislodgement was the important factor. Subsequently, attempts at more appropriate use of drug, schedule, and dose have been subjected to clinical trial by the NSABP (33) and by Bonadonna (34). The preliminary results of both these studies indicate significant improvement in length of disease-free interval especially in premenopausal women. It is too early to be sure that these studies will produce better survival, but these results are encouraging enough to warrant further investigation, and further efforts at improving adjuvant chemotherapy treatments are underway, using combinations of cytotoxic drugs, hormones, and immune stimulating agents.

CONCLUSION

It would appear that extent of surgery is not a determining factor in the successful management of primary breast cancer. Failure, when it occurs, is due to metastases already in place at the time of surgery, and will require systemic therapy, added to adequate local surgery to achieve control adn improve cure rates. Various studies have indicated that radical mastectomy is not more curative than total or simple mastectomy and there is evidence that more conservative surgery, such as segmental mastectomy could achieve equal success. However, conclusive proof of this view is not yet available, due to the lack of adequate trials to test this hypothesis. With present available evidence it would be equally wrong to assume that the case is proven for lesser surgery as it would be to advocate continuing reliance on Radical Mastectomy. Only by completing an appropriate prospective randomized study, such as the ongoing NSABP trial, can a scientific answer be obtained.

REFERENCES

1. Halstead, WS, Results of radical operations for the cure of carcinoma of the breast. Annals Surg 46:1, July, 1907

2. Mc Whirter, R, Simple mastectomy and radiotherapy in treatment of breast cancer. Br J Radiol 28:128, 1955

3. Urban, JA, HW Baker, Radical mastectomy in continuity with en bloc resection of internal mammary lymph-node chain; new procedure for primary operable cancer of breast. Cancer 5:992, 1952

4. Kaae, S, H Johansen, Breast cancer. Comparison of results of simple mastectomy with postoperative roentgen irradiation by McWhirter method with those of extended radical mastectomy. Acta Radiol (Stockh) suppl 188:155, 1959

5. Berkson, J, SW Harrington, OT Clagett, et al, Mortality and survival in surgically treated cancer of breast: statistical summary of some experiences of Mayo Clinic. Proc Mayo Clin 32:645, 1957

6. Paterson, R, MH Russell, Clinical trials in malignant disease - III breast cancer: evaluation of postoperative radiotherapy. J Fac Radiol 10:175, 1959

7. Fisher B, E Montague, C Redmond, et al, Comparison of radical mastectomy with alternative treatments for primary breast cancer. First report of results from prospective randomized clinical trial. Cancer 39 suppl:2827-2839, 1977

8. Fisher, B, The Evolution of Breast Cancer. Seminars in Oncology Vol. 5(4):385-394, December, 1978

9. Spratt, JS, Locally recurrent cancer after radical mastectomy. Cancer 20:1051, 1967

10. Fisher, B, ER Fisher, Interrelationship of hematogenous and lymphatic tumor cell dissemination. Surg Gynecol Obstet 123:791, 1966

11. Fisher, B, N Slack, DL Katrych, et al, Ten year follow-up of breast cancer patients in a cooperative clinical trial evaluating surgical adjuvant chemotherapy. Surg Gynecol Obstet 140:528-534, 1975

12. Mustakallio, S, Treatment of breast cancer by tumor extirpation and roentgen therapy instead of radical operation. J Fac Radiol 6:23, 1954

13. Mustakallio, S, Conservative treatment of breast carcinoma - review of 25 year follow-up. Clin Radiol 23:110, 1972

14. Peters, VM, Wedge resection and irradiation, effective treatment in early breast cancer. JAMA 200:134, 1967

214

15. Wise, L, AY Mason, LV Ackerman, Local excision and irradiation: alternative method for treatment of early mammary cancer. Ann Surg 173:383, 1971

16. Adair, FE, Role of surgery and irradiation in cancer of breast. JAMA 121:553, 1943

17. Porritt, A, Early carcinoma of breast. Br J Surg 51:214, 1964

18. Crile, G, Results of conservative treatment of breast cancer at 10 and 15 years. Ann Surg 182:26, 1975

19. Atkins, H, JL Hayward, DJ Klugman, et al, Treatment of early breast cancer: report after 10 years of clinical trial. Br Med J 2:429, 1972

20. Schabel, FM, Concepts for systemic treatment of micrometastases. Cancer 35:15, 1975

21. Report on an international multicentric trial (1976). Supported by the Cancer Research Campaign. Management of early cancer of the breast. Br Med J 1:1035, 1976

22. Morgenstern, L, PA Kaufman, NB Friedman, Case against tylectomy for carcinoma of breast - factor of multicentricity. Am J Surg 130:251, 1975

23. Crile, G, Multicentric breast cancer: incidence of new cancers in homolateral breast after partial mastectomy. Cancer 35:475, 1975

24. Rosen, PP, AA Fracchia, JA Urban, et al, "Residual" mammary carcinoma following simulated partial mastectomy. Ibid, p 739

25. Fisher, ER, RM Gregoria, B Fisher, et al, Pathology of invasive breast cancer. Syllabus derived from findings of National Surgical Adjuvant Breast Project (protocol #4). Cancer 36:1, 1975

26. Urban JA, Bilateral breast cancer. Cancer 24:1310, 1969

27. Slack, NH, T Nemoto, B Fisher, Experiences with bilateral primary carcinoma of breast. Surg Gynecol Obstet 136:433, 1973

28. McDivitt, RW, RVP Hutter, FW Foote, et al, A prospective follow-up study indicating cumulative patient risks. Lobular Carcinoma 201:96-100, 1967

29. Haagenson, CD, Diseases of Breast. Saunders, Philadelphia, 1966

30. Wheeler, JE, HT Enterline, JM Roseman, JP Tomasulo, CH McIlvaine, WT Fitts, J Kirshenbaum, Lobular cancinoma in situ of the breast. Cancer 34:554-563, 1974

31. Ackerman, LV, AL Katzenstein, The concept of minimal breast cancer and the pathologist's role in the diagnosis of "early carcinoma". Cancer 39:2755-2763, 1977

32. Burchenal, JH, Adjuvant therapy-theory, practice, and potential. Cancer 37:46, 1976

33. Fisher, B, P Carbone, SG Economou, et al, L-phenylalanine mustard (L-PAM) in management of primary breast cancer: report of early findings. N Engl J Med 292:117, 1975

34. Bonadonna G, E Brusamolino, P Valagussa, et al, Combination chemotherapy as adjuvant treatment in operable breast cancer. N Engl J Med 294:405, 1976

CLINICAL APPLICATIONS OF CELL KINETICS TO CHEMOTHERAPY
OF HUMAN MALIGNANCY

Alvin M. Mauer

St. Jude Children's Research Hospital

Memphis, Tennessee

INTRODUCTION

During the past two decades, we have learned a great deal about the characteristics of cell growth in human malignancy. A most important contribution to the study of cell population kinetics was the introduction of the label tritiated thymidine which, for the first time, allowed for the identification of cells in DNA synthesis by autoradiography. Furthermore, in situations where serial samples of the tissue under study could be obtained, it was possible to follow the initially labeled population of DNA synthesizing cells through the subsequent phases of the cell cycle.

It was natural that the initial studies of human malignancy would be done in leukemia because of the ease with which the malignant cells could be sampled from blood and bone marrow. Our basic concepts of cell proliferation in human malignancy were developed from studies of leukemia (1-3).

It is important to briefly review these concepts as necessary background for an understanding of their later application to the design of chemotherapeutic regimens. The leukemia cell populations were found to have a generation cycle longer than their normal cell counterparts: Generation times of 50 to 70 hours, DNA synthesis time of 20 to 25 hours, durations of G_2 and M of about 2 hours each and a minimal time spent in G_1 of 30 to 35 hours. In contrast, normal bone marrow cells have a generation time of about 20 to 25 hours with a DNA synthesis period of about 10 hours. These early studies provided the surprising information that not all leukemic cells were participating in proliferative activity. In fact, in most leukemic cell populations, the growth fraction (that portion of the cell population in the cell cycle) was small, accounting for less than half of the leukemic cells. The growth fraction and the resting cell compartments could be distinguished morphologically by cell size. The resting cells were smaller with denser nuclear chromatin patterns. Through serial studies following labeling with tritiated thymidine, it was possible to demonstrate that cells initially labeled in the growth fraction entered into the resting cell population. Of even greater significance was the demonstration that the resting cells were not end stage cells but were capable of reentry into the growth fraction (4).

216

Considerable variation at diagnosis in the growth fraction from patient to patient was found. It was also demonstrated that variability within the same patient could be found from diagnosis to subsequent relapse. Most frequently, the growth fraction at relapse was greater than at diagnosis. This finding suggested either that proliferative activity was greater during earlier phases of regrowth of a tumor cell population or that with therapy there had been selection of a more actively proliferating subpopulation of the leukemic blasts.

Another important concept growing out of these early studies was the development of evidence for growth regulation of human acute leukemia cell populations (5). This regulation appears to operate through systemic, regional and intrinsic cellular mechanisms (6). From observations of the striking differences in proliferative activity in three different kinds of lymphoid malignancies (common ALL, T cell ALL and B cell lymphoma) it would seem that the most important determining factor for the regulation of proliferative activity is an intrinsic cell characteristic (7). These observations of growth regulation and the observed alterations during phases of the disease set the stage for design of treatment regimens in which deliberate perturbation of proliferative activity were attempted to provide chemotherapeutic advantage.

More recently, the technique of pulse cytophotometry has been added both for the study of leukemic cell populations (8) and solid tumors (9). In this method, the nuclear DNA of the tumor cells is labeled by a fluorescent tag. The amount of label in the nucleus is proportional to the amount of DNA. The labeled cells are subsequently drawn, one at a time, past a laser beam for activation of the fluorescence. The amount of fluorescence given off per cell is measured and by analysis in this manner of a large number of the cells, the distribution by nuclear DNA content can be determined. Subsequent analysis allows the computation of the proportion of cells in various phases of the cell cycle. This technique is rapid and allows for serial determinations of changes occurring in a cell population. The technique has therefore been particularly useful in studying chemotherapeutic perturbation of tumor cell populations.

The concepts described above, developed from studies of human leukemia, have been confirmed for a variety of human solid tumors (10-14). The problems posed for treatment of human cancer can now be much better defined. Clearly, of fundamental importance is the availability of agents more toxic to the tumor cell than for normal cells. Since most agents are maximally effective on a dividing cell, the large resting compartment characteristic of so many human tumors poses the problem of a relatively resistant subpopulation which retains the capability of re-entry into cell proliferation at some future time.

Chemotherapeutic perturbation patterns must be known for optimal drug scheduling, particularly in current treatment schedules in which several agents with differing effects are used. Scheduling must also take into account perturbation of the normal cells. It will be the purpose of the following sections to explore some implications of these findings for the design of treatment programs for human malignancy.

CELL KINETICS AND PROGNOSIS

There has been an attempt to develop a sense of hierarchy among tumor cell populations with respect to initial proliferative activity and responsiveness to therapy. The thesis has been developed that those cancers with the lowest proliferative activity are the most resistant to therapy, while tumors character- ized by large proportions of dividing cells are most sensitive to treatment. In the studies mentioned above of lymphoid malignancies, the common ALL with the least proliferative activity is most responsive to treatment while the increasing proliferative activity found from the T cell leukemia to the B cell lymphoma is associated with a decreasing prognosis for long-term disease-free survival (7). Furthermore, acute lymphocytic leukemia and acute non-lymphocytic leukemia are similar with respect to initial proliferative activity, but clearly different with respect to treatment response (15). Therefore, while there are some reports suggesting prognostic significance of pretreatment proliferative activity in tumor cell populations (16), most studies have not found support for these observations (15, 17). A similar lack of predictability for treatment response has been found in the childhood solid tumor, neuroblastoma (18).

It should be noted, however, that the correlation of initial proliferative activity with response to therapy may be highly treatment dependent. There- fore, in the future, with different treatment regimens, a significant relationship may yet be found.

CHEMOTHERAPEUTIC PERTURBATION OF CELL POPULATION KINETICS

During the past decade, there have been many studies of the perturbation of cell population kinetics by a variety of chemotherapeutic agents (19-27). These studies have been necessary in order to determine the effect of the drugs on malignant cells with respect to phase specificity and the time course of the events. These baseline studies have provided important information with respect to scheduling and the development of combination chemotherapy regimens (28, 29). A summary of these drug effects is given in Table 1.

Table 1. Cell cycle effects of chemotherapeutic agents

Cell cycle phase	Drugs	
	Lethal effects	Progression delay effects
G_1	CCNU, chlorambucil, DTIC, 5-fluorouracil, methotrexate, vinblastine	Actinomycin D, hydrocortisone, 6-mercapto-purine
G_1/S boundary	Actinomycin D, CCNU, methotrexate, nitrogen mustard	Actinomycin D, cytosine arabinoside, 5-fluorouracil, hydrocortisone, methotrexate
S	Adriamycin, L-asparaginase, cytosine arabinoside, daunomycin, DTIC, 5-fluorouracil, methotrexate, vinblastine, vincristine	DTIC
S/G_2 boundary	Adriamycin	Actinomycin D, cytosine arabinoside
A_2	5-fluorouracil, VM26	Actinomycin D, adriamycin, CCNU, cyclo-phosphamide, daunomycin, nitrogen mustard, VM26
M	Actinomycin D, adriamycin, CCNU, chlorambucil, 5-fluorouracil, nitrogen mustard, vinblastine	Vinblastine, vincristine

Modified from Hill T and Baserga, The cell cycle and its significance for cancer treatment. Cancer Treat Rev 2:159, 1975
CCNU = Cis-cyclohexyl nitrosourea; DTIC: dimethyl triazeno imidazole carbox amide

From these studies of single agents, it was evident that the tumor cell population could be perturbed by cell cycle synchronization and recruitment of resting cells (30-37). Attempts at synchronization take advantage of the effects of some drugs to delay cells in their passage through some phase of the cell cycle. As examples, cytosine arabinoside delays cells in DNA synthesis and small doses of vincristine can delay cells in mitosis. As cells continue to enter the delayed phase, there is a progressive accumulation; and if the drug effect is temporary, subsequent release of these cells allows for progression through the cell cycle in a partially synchronized manner. The purpose of synchronization is to introduce a second agent which is phase specific for cytotoxicity at a time of greatest accumulation of delayed cells. Enhancement of the effectiveness of the second agent is sought by increasing the number of sensitive cells. In human malignancy, the greatest problem has been variability in the degree of synchronization obtained and the timing of greatest accumulation. This variability has meant that each patient must be monitored for the appropriate timing of the second agent. This need has made the application of cell cycle synchronization to large clinical trials currently a virtual impossibility.

Recruitment of resting cells into the cell cycle has also been observed following chemotherapeutic perturbation. The mechanism is presumed to be the reduction of tumor cell mass calling into play growth control mechanisms which increase tumor cell proliferative activity. An alternative possibility would be the chemotherapy-induced selection of subpopulations of tumor cells having the greater degree of proliferative activity. Unfortunately, there are few human tumor cell systems in which it is possible to make simultaneous measurements of tumor cell mass and proportion of proliferating cells to make a true measurement of recruitment (38). Recruitment in most situations must be inferential (18). More fundamental knowledge of the growth regulation of tumor cell populations and the possibility of subpopulation selection by chemotherapy will no doubt be necessary to take full advantage of this mechanism of enhancement of chemotherapeutic advantage.

SCHEDULING FOR NORMAL AND TUMOR CELL RESPONSE

Not only is it important to schedule chemotherapy regimens for maximal tumoricidal effect, but it is also important to spare to the greatest degree possible the normal dividing cell populations, especially in bone marrow and digestive tract mucosa. Information concerning the effects of cancer chemotherapeutic agents on normal hematopoietic precursor cells is becoming available (39). Of particular importance is the increasing number of studies in which there has been simultaneous evaluation of the kinetic response of normal and malignant tissues (40-42). The major aim of these studies is to get information concerning the relative rates of recovery of normal and tumor cell populations following the administration of a drug. The time of maximal sensitivity of a cell population to the administration of a second agent is the period of greatest proliferative activity following recovery. In general, the normal cell population's return of proliferative activity precedes that of the tumor cell population. Avoiding the maximal proliferative activity of normal cells, and giving the second dose while normal cells are in steady state and tumor cells are recovering, provides an important therapeutic advantage. Unfortunately, in some tumors, recovery of the normal and cancer cells occurs simultaneously so that timing of the second dose for maximal effect on tumor cells also results in maximal toxicity. The variability observed in studies so far would indicate the need to monitor proliferative changes in patients in which this form of scheduling is being attempted.

A real advantage for treatment of cancer would be obtained if it were possible to have an early prediction for nonresponding tumors. If it were possible to identify those patients who would not respond to a treatment regimen, then alternative therapy could be promptly begun. This opportunity would avoid the needless toxicity of an ineffective regimen and more promptly shift the patient to an alternative regimen without the delay of waiting for obvious lack of clinical response. Some recent studies have demonstrated a correlation of changes in the cell kinetic patterns with response to treatment (18, 43-45). Further studies of the relationship of chemotherapeutic perturbation of cell kinetic patterns and response to therapy are needed. If a consistent relationship can be demonstrated, this approach might also be most valuable for the more rapid evaluation of the effectiveness of new agents. Certainly, the current method of measuring clinical response in Phase II studies requires lengthy observation and exposure to a potentially ineffective but toxic agent.

SUMMARY

Within the relatively brief time of two decades, there has been a considerable conceptual advance concerning human tumor cell proliferation. Within the past decade, there likewise has been learned a great deal about the effects of chemotherapeutic agents on the proliferation of both normal and cancer cells. Attempts at using this information to devise better treatment schedules have been made difficult by the variability in responses observed. With the availability of the pulse cytophotometer and its ability to provide prompt information concerning changes in cell cycle distribution, individualized treatment schedules might be possible. Observations of the relationship of cell cycle changes and response to therapy need to be extended for their possible usefulness in predicting response in the individual patient as well as adjunct in evaluating new drugs. There is also a need for more information on the relative changes induced in normal and cancer cell populations to assist in scheduling drug administration in order to avoid toxicity.

ACKNOWLEDGEMENT
This work was supported by Core Grant CA21765, and by ALSAC.

REFERENCES

1. Gavasto, F, A Pileri, V Gabutti, and P Masera, Cell population kinetics in human acute leukaemia. Europ J Cancer 3:301-307, 1967

2. Killmann, SA, Acute leukemia: The kinetics of leukemic blast cells in man. Ser Haemat 1:38-102, 1968

3. Mauer, AM, BC Lampkin, Studies of leukemia cell proliferation. In: Advances in Acute Leukemia, Cleton, FJ, D Crowther, and SS Malpas (eds), North Holland Publishing Co, Amsterdam, 1:69-94, 1974

4. Saunders, EF and AM Mauer, Reentry of nondividing leukemic cells into a proliferative phase in acute childhood leukemia. J Clin Invest 48:1299-1305, 1969

5. Mauer, AM and SB Murphy, Growth regulation of human acute leukemia cell populations. In: Proceedings of a Symposium - Fundamental Aspects of Neoplasia, Gottlieb, AA (ed), Springer-Verlag, New York, p 389-399, 1975

6. Mauer AM, SB Murphy, and FA Hayes, Growth regulations of human malignant cells. In: Results and Problems in Cell Differentiation, Berrmann W, WJ Gehring, JB Gurdon, FC Kafatos, and J Reinert (eds), Springer-Verlag, Inc, New York (in press)

7. Murphy, SB, SL Melvin, and AM Mauer, Correlation of tumor cell kinetic studies with surface marker results in childhood non-Hodgkin's lymphoma. Cancer Res 39:1534-1538, 1979

8. Hillen, H, J Wessels, and C Hannen, Bone-marrow proliferation patterns in acute myeloblastic leukemia determined by pulse cytophotometry. Lancet i:609-614, 1975

9. Barlogie, B, W Gohde, DA Johnston, L Smallwood, et al, Determination of ploidy and proliferative characteristics of human solid tumors by pulse cytophotometry. Cancer Res 38:3333-3339, 1978

10. Young, RC and VT DeVita, Cell cycle characteristics of human solid tumors in vivo. Cell Tissue Kinet 3:285-290, 1970

11. Sullivan, PW and SE Salmon, Kinetics of tumor growth and regression in IgG multiple myeloma. J Clin Invest 51:1697-1708, 1972

12. Hainau, B and P Dombernowsky, Histology and cell proliferation in human bladder tumors. Cancer 33:115-126, 1974

13. Muggia, FM, SK Krezoski, and HH Hansen, Cell kinetic studies in patients with small cell carcinoma of the lung. Cancer 34:1683-1690, 1974

224

14. Terz, JJ, W Lawrence, Jr, and B Cox, Analysis of the cycling and non-cycling cell population of human solid tumors. Cancer 40:1462-1470, 1977

15. Murphy, AM, RJA Aur, JV Simone, S George, and AM Mauer, Pretreatment cytokinetic studies in 94 children with acute leukemia. Relationship to other variables at diagnosis and to outcome of standard treatment. Blood 49:683-691, 1977

16. Hart, JS, SL George, E Frei, III, GP Bodey, et al, Prognostic significance of pretreatment proliferative activity in adult acute leukemia. Cancer 39:1603-1617, 1977

17. Amadori, S, MC Petti, A DeFrancesco, A Chierichini, et al, Lack of prognostic significance of the pretreatment labeling and mitotic indices of marrow blasts in acute nonlymphocytic leukemia (ANLL). Cancer 41:1154-1160, 1978

18. Hayes, FA, AA Green, and AM Mauer, Correlation of cell kinetic and clinical response to chemotherapy in disseminated neuroblastoma. Cancer Res 37:3766-3770, 1977

19. Lampkin, BC, T Nagao, and AM Mauer, Drug effect in acute leukemia. J Clin Invest 48:1124-1130, 1969

20. Ernst, P and SA Killmann, Perturbation of generation cycle of human leukemia blast cells by cytostatic therapy in vivo: Effect of corticosteroids. Blood 36:689-696, 1970

21. Ernst, P and SA Killmann, Perturbation of generation cycle of human leukemic myeloblasts in vivo by methotrexate. Blood 38:689-705, 1971

22. Howell, SB, A Krishan, and E Frei, III, Cytokinetic comparison of thymidine and leucovorin rescue of marrow in humans after exposure to high-dose methotrexate. Cancer Res 39:1315-1320, 1979

23. Barlogie, B, B. Drewinki, DA Johnston, and EJ Freireich, III, The effect of adriamycin on the cell cycle traverse of a human lymphoid cell line. Cancer Res 36:1975-1979, 1976

24. Ernst, P, A Faille, and SA Killmann, Perturbation of cell cycle of human leukemic myeloblasts in vivo by cytosine arabinoside. Scand J Haemat 10:209-218, 1973

25. Yataganas, X, A Strife, A Perez, and BD Clarkson, Microbluorimetric evaluation of cell kill kinetics with 1 - β -D - arabinofuranosylcytosine. Cancer Res 34:2795-2806, 1974

26. Krishnan, A, K Paika, and E Frei, III, Cytofluorometric studies on the action of podophyllotoxinand epipodophyllotoxins (VM - 26, VP - 16 - 213) on the cell cycle traverse of human lymphoblasts. J Cell Biol 66:521-530, 1975.

27. Wagner, HP, PM Swidzinska, and A Hirt, Variable duration of vincristine-induced metaphase block in leukemic and normal bone marrow cells of children. Med Pediatr Oncol 3:75-83, 1977

28. Lampkin, BC, NB McWilliams, and AM Mauer, Cell kinetics and chemotherapy in acute leukemia. Semin Hematol 9:211-223, 1972

29. Valeriote, F and L van Putten, Proliferation-dependent cytotoxicity of anticancer agents: A review. Cancer Res 35:2619-2630, 1975

30. Lampkin, BC, T Nagao, and AM Mauer, Synchronization of the mitotic cycle in acute leukemia. Nature 222:1274-1275, 1969

31. Lampkin, BC, T Nagao, and AM Mauer, Synchronization and recruitment in acute leukemia. J Clin Invest 50:2204-2214, 1971

32. Pouillart P, R Weiner, L Schwarzenberg, JL Misset, et al, Med Pediatr Oncol 1:123-134, 1975

33. Vogler, WR, WB Kremer, WH Knospe, GA Omura, et al, Synchronization with phase-specific agents in leukemia and correlation with clinical response to chemotherapy. Cancer Treat Rep 60:1845-1859, 1976

34. Klein, HO, KJ Lennartz, R Gross, M Eder, et al, In-vivo und in-vitro untersuchungen zur zellkinetic und synchronisation menschlicher tumorzellen. Dtsch Med Wochenschr 97:1273-1282, 1972

35. Burke, PJ and AH Owens, Jr, Attempted recruitment of leukemic myeloblasts to proliferative activity by sequential drug treatment. Cancer 28:830-836, 1971

36. Burke, PJ, JE Karp, HG Braine, and WP Vaughan, Timed sequential therapy of human leukemia based upon the response of leukemic cells to humoral growth factors. Cancer Res 37:2138-2146, 1977

37. Karp, JE and PJ Burke, Enhancement of drug cytotoxicity by recruitment of leukemic myeloblasts with humoral stimulation. Cancer Res 36:3600-3603, 1976

38. Salmon, SE, Expansion of the growth fraction in multiple myeloma with alkylating agents. Blood 45:119-129, 1975

39. Marsh, JC, The effects of cancer chemotherapeutic agents on normal hematopoietic precursor cells: A review. Cancer Res 36:1853-1882, 1976

226

40. Rosenoff, SH, JM Bull, and RC Young, The effect of chemotherapy on the kinetics and proliferative capacity of normal and tumorous tissues in vivo. Blood 45:107-117, 1975

41. Rosenoff, SH, F Bostick, and RC Young, Recovery of normal hematopoietic tissue and tumor following chemotherapeutic injury from cyclophosphamide (CTX): Comparative analysis of biochemical and clinical techniques. Blood 45:465-475, 1975

42. Myers, CE, RC Young, and BA Chabner, Kinetic alterations induced by 5-fluorouracil in bone marrow, intestinal mucosa, and tumor. Cancer Res 36:1653-1658, 1976

43. Vogler, WR, LE Cooper, and DP Groth, Correlation of cytosine arabinoside-induced increment in growth fraction of leukemic blast cells with clinical response. Cancer 33:603-610, 1974

44. Zittoun, R, M Bouchard, J Facquet-Danis, M Percie-Du-Sert, and J Bousser, Prediction of the response to chemotherapy in acute leukemia. Cancer 35:507-513, 1975

45. Murphy, WK, RB Livingston, VG Ruiz, FG Gercovich, et al, Serial labeling index determination as a predictor of response in human solid tumors. Cancer Res 35:1438-1444, 1975

ADJUVANT THERAPY IN CHILDHOOD
NEOPLASMS - AN OVERVIEW

W.W. Sutow

The University of Texas System Cancer Center,

M. D. Anderson Hospital and Tumor Institute

Houston, Texas

INTRODUCTION

Dr. Frank M. Schabel, Jr. has outlined the fascinating fundamental concepts of neoplastic cell growth and cell kill based on data that have emerged from his studies in the laboratory in collaboration with Howard E. Skipper and colleagues (1).

This presentation will be a report of what is happening on the human front in the war against cancer. It shall be the intent to indicate the state of the art, clinically, in respect to treatment and control of certain malignant solid tumors of childhood. It is emphasized that many of the current techniques of multidisciplinary and adjuvant therapy were pioneered and developed in pediatric oncology - against childhood cancer. Accordingly, it is pertinent to review, in perspective, how we got where we are. Further, certain significant landmarks must be defined for orientation. Lastly, some speculations can be made regarding projections the current achievements may justifiably permit (2).

As the leading medical cause of death today in children 1 through 14 years of age, cancer is a major pediatric problem. Yet, numerically, the incidence of cancer in children is minute, compared to the adults. Based on the Third National Cancer Survey (3) conducted in 1969, 1970 and 1971, and related to the National Census of 1970, the most accurate estimate of the incidence of cancer in children has been made available recently (4). The occurrence of cancer of all types in children was calculated to be 124 per million among white children and 97 per million among black children. Solid tumors accounted for 55% of all cancer. The five most frequent solid tumors were, in order, brain tumors, neuroblastoma, rhabdomyosarcoma, Wilms' tumor and bone tumor (table 1).

Table 1

RELATIVE FREQUENCY OF SOLID TUMORS
IN CHILDHOOD CANCER

Brain tumors	35%
Neuroblastoma	14
Rhabdomyosarcoma	12
Wilms' tumor	11
Bone cancer	8
Retinoblastoma	5
Miscellaneous	15

Three of these solid tumors (Wilms' tumor, rhabdomyosarcoma) and osteosarcoma will exemplify the nature of the clinical problems, the strategies utilized and the results of current multimodal programs.

WILMS' TUMOR

Early Studies

By 1945 to 1950, the first plateau (at about 35% to 40%) was being approached in treatment results measured as long-term survival rates for Wilms' tumor (5-7). By that time, the surgical techniques had been well established. The importance of postoperative (postnephrectomy) radiation therapy had also been recognized. Postoperative supportive care and anesthetic procedures had been refined and expanded. There was, however, no effective adjuvant chemotherapy regimen.

In the early fifties, Sidney Farber at Boston performed pioneer work in the administration of actinomycin D as adjuvant to surgery and radiation in the overall primary management of Wilms' tumor (5,8). In the early sixties a second effective drug, vincristine, became available. The drug was useful in the treatment of metastatic Wilms' tumor (9), and its value as adjuvant chemotherapy was established early (10). The drug appeared to be effective as preoperative chemotherapy in order to facilitate the surgical procedures (11). Most recently, in the present decade of the seventies, a third drug, Adriamycin, has shown significant antitumor activity (12). Its potential usefulness and place in the general approach to Wilms' tumor are currently being assessed. The net result of all these developments has been the progressive improvement in the survival curves for children with this tumor (6,7,13).

National Wilms' Tumor Study Group

One of the major forces that have changed the clinical attitudes toward Wilms' tumor has been the collaborative investigations monitored by the National Wilms' Tumor Study (NWTS) Committee (14). Basic and significant findings are emerging from these national studies. The concepts for NWTS were generated about 1966 but the actual study (NWTS-1) did not become functional until 1969.

One of the initial approaches was the adoption of the clinical grouping schema (14,15). The term "group" was used, instead of the term "stage". The purpose was to indicate the extent of the disease (clinical, surgical and pathological) at the start of therapy. It differed in definition from the usual concept of "stage" because the end result of the definitive surgical procedure was taken into consideration (see table 2).

Table 2

CLINICAL GROUPING SCHEMA UTILIZED
IN NWTS-1 AND NWTS-2 (15,18)

Clinical Group	Definition
I	Tumor limited to kidney and completely resected.
II	Tumor extends regionally beyond kidney but is completely resected.
III	Residual non-hematogenous tumor confined to abdomen.
IV	Hematogenous metastases.
V	Bilateral renal involvement either initially or subsequently.

NWTS-1

Analysis of NWTS-1 validated the concept of clinical grouping. The outcome of therapy (prognosis) was significantly correlated with clinical group (14). Other aspects of NWTS have also made significant impacts on pediatric oncology.

In Group I patients where the tumor was localized to the kidney and was completely excised, the NWTS-1 addressed this question: In such patients, was postoperative irradiation of the tumor bed necessary? All Group I patients eligible for the study underwent nephrectomy and received actinomycin D as chemotherapy. One half of the patients were then given radiotherapy. The other half of the patients received no postoperative irradiation. Statistical analysis showed that all Group I patients had exceedingly good chances for survival - over 90%. The curves for those receiving irradiation and those not receiving irradiation showed no difference statistically (14). From these data it was concluded that in Group I patients, the omission of postoperative irradiation of the tumor beds resulted in no catastrophic outcome.

In Group II and III patients, it was assumed that the tumor was more extensive so that it had a greater potential for local recurrence or distant spread. In these patients, a different question was asked in NWTS-1. There were two chemotherapeutic agents known to be effective against Wilms' tumor - actinomycin D and vincristine. Which drug was better? Or was the combination of the two drugs more effective than either alone? All patients had nephrectomy. Postoperative irradiation was given to all. Randomly, one-third of the patients received actinomycin D alone as the adjuvant chemotherapy; one-third received vincristine only; and the final one-third received both actinomycin D and vincristine. When survival data were analyzed, it was found that:

(1) Those receiving vincristine alone did as well as those receiving actinomycin D alone;

(2) However, those receiving both drugs had a significantly superior survival than either of the other two sets of patients.

The results, therefore, permitted the conclusionthat in Group II and III patients, the combination of vincristine and actinomycin D was a more effective adjuvant chemotherapy program than vincristine alone or actinomycin D alone. Clinically, these results meant that all Group II and III patients should be treated at least with both drugs.

One of the surprising results of NWTS-1 concerned bilateral Wilms' tumor. In 5% of the cases (30 out of about 600), the tumor involved the second kidney, either at the time of diagnosis or subsequently (16). Although these cases were treated individually by the investigators, the outcome appeared unusually good.

The projected survival in these 30 cases was 87% at 2+ years. These early findings were most encouraging, but the 5 year survival data would be more definitive. Another result of the first NWT study was the observation that the histopathology of Wilms' tumor could indicate good prognosis or bad prognosis (17). A detailed examination of the first 300 diagnostic slides that had been forwarded to the study showed that the histopathology could be divided into 2 groups. Approximately 12% showed anaplastic or rhabdomyosarcomatous pattern. The other 88% contained differentiated renal structures. When the histologic divisions were correlated with prognosis, a significant difference was noted. About a third of the group with differentiated histopathology had died. In contrast, 95% of the smaller group were dead. Subsequently, the terms favorable and unfavorable have been used to designate these two histologic categories.

NWTS-2*

On the basis of results from the first national study, the second study (NWTS-2) is currently underway (18). In stage I patients, postoperative radiotherapy is not given. The question concerns the duration of chemotherapy required for optimum results. Both actinomycin D and vincristine are used. On a random basis, one-half will be given the drugs for 6 months and the other one-half will receive both drugs for 15 months as in the first study. In stages II, III and IV, more effective therapy is still needed. Consequently, a random one-half will be given both vincristine and actinomycin D for 15 months in addition to post-operative therapy. The regimen is the same as that used in the first study. The other one-half will be treated in the same manner except that Adriamycin has been added. This will be therefore a comparison between a 2-drug and a 3-drug regimen.

To summarize, the score regarding Wilms' tumor at the present time reads as follows:

(a) Over 90% of Group I patients should remain disease free and the overall long term survival rate should be over 95%.

(b) The overall longterm survival when all stage I, II and III patients are combined should be over 70%.

(c) Even in patients who fail in initial therapy, the salvage rate is estimated to be approaching 40%.

*The preliminary results of NWTS-2 was abstracted In Proc: AACR & ASCO 20:309, 1979.

The goals of current approaches to the handling of patients with Wilms' tumor would include the following:

(1) The question of optimal postoperative radiotherapy should be examined continuously. As the effectiveness of chemotherapy improves, the required intensity of radiation therapy should decrease. As already demonstrated in Group I patients, the ultimate elimination of radiation therapy in other clinical groups would be ideal.

(2) The question of optimal chemotherapy in terms of the nature of the drug combinations, the drug sequence and schedule, and the duration of therapy needs further investigation.

(3) Methods to improve the survival of those who fail on primary therapy have to be investigated.

(4) Now that histopathology can be correlated with prognosis, there is recognized the urgent need to plug this vital information meaningfully into the management strategy.

(5) The unexpectedly good results documented in patients with bilateral Wilms' tumor emphasize the viable possibility that treatment programs for these patients could be systematically planned and studied.

(6) In addition, the surviving children will reach adulthood and have children of their own. The genetic implications of this tumor in respect to offspring, sibs and relatives of the patients must be studied (19,20).

(7) With improved survival, the occurrence of late deleterious effects of therapy become a significant consideration (21,22).

RHABDOMYOSARCOMA

Background

Childhood rhabdomyosarcoma is another malignant solid tumor of major importance in pediatric oncology since it is relatively frequent. This tumor is responsive to intensive therapy, and the significant part of this partial success occurred in the past 10 to 15 years. The drugs found to be most effective against this tumor include vincristine, actinomycin D, and cyclophosphamide. Methotrexate, however, even in massive doses in conjunction with citrovorum factor, has not shown significant antitumor activity. Although Adriamycin appears to have some effect on the tumor, the degree of this activity needs to be further established.

In 1965, a 3-drug combination of vincristine, actinomycin D and cyclophosphamide, acronymically called VAC, yielded some impressive results (23). A survival rate of greater than 60%, was achieved with VAC combined with radiotherapy in a group of children with rhabdomyosarcoma of the head and neck (24,25). In almost all of them, surgery was not possible. (Orbital cases were excluded).

Intergroup Rhabdomyosarcoma Study

In 1972, a national study of rhabdomyosarcoma, the Intergroup Rhabdomyosarcoma Study (IRS), was activated (26,27). Patterned after the Wilms' Tumor Study, the extent of the disease was assessed on the basis of demonstrable disease and the result of initial surgical procedure. The grouping system was then utilized to determine therapy. The results of the interim analysis of the data (27,28) indicate that the grouping system was valid - when measured in terms of disease free survival. Group I patients show an impressive survival of about 85% at 3 years. Group II patients have 3 year survival around 70%. Group III patients plateau at about 55%. Group IV patients do poorly, with only about 10% surviving at 3 years.

In the IRS, all Group I patients received the standard VAC therapy. One-half of the patients were randomized to receive, in addition, radiotherapy to the tumor bed. The other half received no irradiation. Results show that in terms of the disease free rate, frequency of local recurrence, or survival, there is no difference between the two arms of the study. Thus, it is concluded that in Group I patients, the omission of radiotherapy has no influence on treatment outcome.

In Group II patients, the tumor locally is more extensive than in Group I patients. All Group II patients therefore received irradiation to the tumor bed. A random one-half of the patients received the standard VAC chemotherapy. In the other one-half, cyclophosphamide was omitted. These patients received only vincristine and actinomycin D. The results show that there is no difference in the disease free rate or in survival between the group that received VAC and the group that received only vincristine and actinomycin D. It is concluded that in Group II patients the two-drug combination (VCR + AMD) seems to be equally effective as three drugs (VCR + AMD + CYT). Being able to omit cyclophosphamide from the treatment regimen without loss of effectiveness would be a big advantage. The acute and late toxicity of cyclophosphamide can thus be avoided.

In Group III patients where residual gross tumor is present, and in Group IV patients where metastases have occurred, the effort was made to compare the standard 3-drug regimen with a 4-drug regimen in which Adriamycin was added to VAC. The purpose was to intensify the chemotherapy. The results show no difference in results in the Group III patients between regimen E (which was the standard VAC treatment) and regimen F (which included Adriamycin). The disease free rate at 3 years was less than 60%. In group IV patients, again there is also no significant difference between patients receiving 3-drugs (regimen E) and those receiving 4-drugs (regimen F). At 3 years the survival rate is less than 20%.

The IRS also confirmed the earlier clinical experience that the site of the primary appeared to influence prognosis using the treatment available at this time: genitourinary cases had the best survival and extremity cases the poorest survival. Head and neck cases had intermediate survival statistics.

On the basis of the findings from the first study (27-29), the protocol for a second national study in rhabdomyosarcoma has been finalized.[*] A brief review of the proposed second study may serve to point out some of the current goals. In Group I patients no radiotherapy is given. One group will be randomized to receive 2-drugs, VCR and AMD. The other group will receive standard VAC therapy. The purpose here is to test the possibility that Group I patients do not need radiation therapy and may also not need cyclophosphamide.

In Group II patients, the comparison will be between a 2-drug regimen of VCR and AMD and a 3-drug VAC regimen given on a different schedule - that is, as intermittent pulses. There is some clinical experience that suggests that the intermittent schedule is more effective and less toxic. In Group III and Group IV patients, the second Intergroup Study proposes to compare the intermittent pulse VAC regimen with an intensified 4-drug regimen that includes Adriamycin.

Planning For Special Sites. The results from IRS-1 also demonstrated a major problem area. This concerned patients with primary tumors situated in parameningeal sites (31). The parameningeal sites were considered to be nasopharynx, nasal cavity, nasal sinuses and middle ear. There were 57 patients with parameningeal primary tumors. In 20 of these patients (35%), the disease eventually involved the central nervous system. Once there was CNS extension,

*IRS-2 was activated in November, 1978. See reference (30) for most current report of results.

of the CNS problems that once complicated treatment of children with acute leukemia (32). In the second IRS, therefore, it is proposed to attack this potential danger prophylactically. All patients with primary lesion in paramenin-geal sites will be evaluated carefully. Of particular importance are the assessment of bone erosion at the base of brain and examination of the CSF. If the findings are considered to be negative, there will be no change in chemotherapy. The radiotherapy fields will be carefully checked to insure a 2-cm margin about the tumor. If, however, the initial evaluation is considered to be positive, a program of craniospinal irradiation and intrathecal chemotherapy will be carried out.

It has been mentioned that patients with GU rhabdomyosarcoma had unusually good survival rates. However, in many cases, survival was achieved at the cost of an extensive mutilating type of surgery such as pelvic exenteration. In IRS-2 the possibility of changing this approach is being evaluated. Therefore, patients with pelvic rhabdomyosarcoma (that is, the patients with primary tumors involving the bladder, prostate and vulvo-vagina) will be handled separately. These patients will receive primary chemotherapy (that is, preoperative chemotherapy). Two courses of pulse-VAC are given. The clinical status is evaluated by the pediatric oncologist and by the surgeon (urologist or gynecologist) at week 8. At that time it is determined whether a) the disease has shown partial or complete regression or b) the disease has shown no response or is progressive, (that is, there is increasing disease). If there is complete or partial regression at week 8, chemotherapy is continued for 8 more weeks. At week 16, definitive surgery is carried out. It is hoped that a less than radical surgery can be used and that exenteration can be avoided. No postoperative radiation therapy is planned if the tumor can be completely resected. If there is residual tumor postoperatively, then radiation therapy will have to be employed.

OSTEOSARCOMA

Background

Osteosarcoma is a primary cancer of the bone which occurs predominantly in the young between 10 and 30 years of age. It is also a tumor that had been considered to be radioresistant and chemoresistant. For decades, the survival rate had been consistently low. Regardless of the treatment used, the survival in all large series was less than 20% and in many, considerably below 20% (34). It would seem reasonable to assume, therefore, that a patient in whom a diagnosis of osteosarcoma is made, has an 80 to 90% probability that he has already either demonstrable or occult microscopic metastases. It is a tumor in which the primary lesion can be effectively and completely removed by amputation. Thus any change in the survival pattern must be attibuted to treatment that is instituted after or in addition to the surgical removal of the primary tumor, i.e. surgical adjuvant therapy.

Adjuvant Chemotherapy

Adjuvant chemotherapy is defined here as treatment used in a patient with osteosarcoma who has no demonstrable evidence of disease other than the primary tumor. The primary tumor is extirpated surgically (generally and until recently, by amputation). The chronology of the evolution of the adjuvant chemotherapy program for osteosarcoma at M. D. Anderson Hospital will illustrate the recognition and introduction of various drugs into the program at different times (table 3) (35). A single agent approach using phenylalanine mustard (PAM) was started in 1962. The results from this initial PAM study were unimpressive. Among 14 patients treated with PAM there was no improvement in survival over the general experience. In 1969 VAC was evaluated as adjuvant therapy, primarily because of the very good results which were being seen in childhood rhabdomyosarcoma with the VAC regimen (23). The results from the pulse-VAC regimen were most encouraging. Among 12 children treated, 4 or 33% remained disease free (35).

About that time, the Adriamycin data became available (36). PAM, VAC and Adriamycin were therefore combined into the 4-drug program acronymically designated as CONPADRI-I (about 1970). The drugs were given in several combinations on a schedule determined by patient tolerance over a period of 54 weeks. In the first 18 patients treated, 10 have remained disease free - a survival rate of 55% (37). These patients are now all 6 years and longer from time of diagnosis. With the demonstration that HD-MTX was effective in metastatic osteosarcoma (38), MTX was added to CONPADRI-I, making the new program a 5-drug combination (COMPADRI-II) in 1972. Since then there has been a progressive modification of the combination to formulate COMPADRI-V. In general, the modifications were intended to make the treatment more effective by increasing the dose and by increasing the frequency, generally, of the methotrexate courses.

In COMPADRI-II and COMPADRI-III, the methotrexate was used at the front-end. The results have been somewhat disappointing. Because of late relapses, particularly with COMPADRI-II, the survival curves appear to be no better than the curve for CONPADRI-I. COMPADRI-III was intensified first by increasing the frequency of HD-MTX pulses. The MTX-pulses consist of two doses given a week apart. Three pulses are given during the first 9 weeks (or 6 doses of HD-MTX). Second, the total number of pulses were increased, and third, the doses for MTX and Adriamycin were also increased. Most recently, the adjuvant program has been modified again to COMPADRI-V. This was done to adapt the chemotherapy regimen to increasing interest in limb salvage procedures and to minimize the delay of chemotherapy in many patients because of surgery.

Schematically, in COMPADRI-V the diagnosis is made within 24 to 48 hours after initial visit, in almost all cases through a needle biopsy. HD-MTX pulses I, and II, a week apart, are started. There is a 5 week rest period. Then pulses III and IV, again a week apart, are given. Definitive surgery is done about week 6. The second phase consists of Adriamycin. During the third phase, additional chemotherapy is given through week 54. On the basis of available data, the current capabilities in managing patients with osteosarcoma can be projected to provide disease-free survival at this time, in 50 to 70% of the patients presenting with non-metastatic disease (39). The overall survival should be even better. The data at M.D. Anderson Hospital show that in patients under 20 years of age with extremity lesions, the 3-year survival rate is 79% (40).

Much has been accomplished in the management of osteosarcoma, but further work still remains to be performed. With respect to future goals and current activity in the management of osteosarcoma, the following areas need to be considered:

(1) There is still need to improve the efficacy of treatment. Late relapses have occurred in practically all series treated at various centers. The potential combination of chemotherapy with radiation therapy still needs additional evaluation.

(2) The potential and the applicability of limb-salvage procedures are being evaluated in many centers. Surgical excision of tumor with prosthetic replacement are being successfully achieved with functional limb preservation.

(3) Increasingly aggressive surgical, radiotherapeutic and chemotherapeutic modalities are being combined to achieve longterm survival even after the development of metastases.

Table 3

DEVELOPMENT OF MULTIDRUG ADJUVANT CHEMOTHERAPY FOR OSTEOSARCOMA

M.D. ANDERSON HOSPITAL (34)

Time Period	Drug (s)	Principles(s) Tested and Results Obtained
1960-1971	Phenylalanine mustard (PAM)	Determination of antitumor activity of PAM used singly against osteosarcoma; antitumor activity (temporary) noted from 10% (2/19) to 43% (3/7) of patients with metastases.
1962-1968	PAM	Use as adjuvant chemotherapy in patients with nonmetastatic osteosarcoma; disease-free survival rate of 14% (2/14) achieved.
1969-1971	Pulse-VAC (vincristine, actinomycin-D, cyclophosphamide)	Utilization of VAC regimen effective in another tumor (rhabdomyosarcoma) as adjuvant therapy in osteosarcoma; disease-free survival rate of 33% (4/12) achieved.
1970-1972	Adriamycin	Evaluation of reported antitumor activity of Adriamycin in metastatic osteosarcoma; antitumor activity (temporary) documented in about 40% (5/13) of patients with metastases.
1970-1975	CONPADRI-I	Adjuvant chemotherapy with four-drug combination (cyclophosphamide, vincristine, PAM, and Adriamycin); long-term disease-free rate of 55% (10/18) achieved; similar disease-free rate obtained in expanded SWOG Group study (24/44).

1972-	High-dose methotrexate	Evaluation of reported antitumor activity in metastatic osteosarcoma of high-dose methotrexate with citrovorum factor; antitumor activity (temporary) reported in about 85% (6/7) of patients with metastases.
1973-1977	COMPADRI-II-IV	Addition of HD-MTX to CONPADRI-I; extensive pharmacokinetic studies of HD-MTX and development of systems for pharmacologic monitoring; intensification of HD-MTX and Adriamycin schedules to combat late metastases; long-term disease-free survival rate in COMPADRI-II and III (27/60) and (22/44) less than in CONPADRI-I; follow-up date from COMPADRI-IV still too early for analysis.
1977	COMPADRI-V	Intensification of HD-MTX and Adriamycin dose/schedule; "front-loading" concept; preoperative chemotherapy; "limb-salvage" surgical approaches; pilot studies well underway.

(4) One of the precepts of surgical treatment of osteosarcoma has been the complete removal of the entire bone involved with tumor. With chemotherapy it is possible that transmedullary amputation (that is, amputation through the involved bone) may become more widespread. The presence of a stump greatly facilitates the use of prostheses.

(5) In some circumstances, is it possible to think about prophylactic therapy? Considerations along that line requires that the population at risk must be identified and the magnitude of the risk must be assessed. Such populations include survivors of retinoblastoma (20), particularly those with bilateral retinoblastoma, and survivors of Ewing's sarcoma treated with radiotherapy (41).

REFERENCES

1. Schabel, FM, Jr, Experimental basis for adjuvant chemotherapy, In: Adjuvant Therapy of Cancer, Salmon SE and Jones SE, (eds), Elsevier/North-Holland Biomedical Press, Amsterdam, 1977, p 345-356

2. Sutow, WW, Adjuvant therapy in Wilms' tumor, rhabdomyosarcoma, osteosarcoma and other childhood neoplasms - an overview. In: Adjuvant Therapy of Cancer, Salmon, SE and Jones SE, (eds), Elsevier/North-Holland Biomedical Press, Amsterdam, 1977, p 345-356

3. Cutler SJ and JL Young Jr, (eds), The third national cancer survey: Incidence data. Nat'l Cancer Inst Monographs 41:1-454, 1975

4. Young, JL, Jr, and RW Miller, Incidence of malignant tumors in U.S. children. J Pediatr 86:254-258, 1975

5. Farber, S, Chemotherapy in the treatment of leukemia and Wilms' tumor. JAMA 198:826-836, 1966

6. Sutow, WW, Wilms' tumor - retrospect and prospect. Proc Am Cancer Soc Nat'l Conf on the Care of the Child with Cancer. George F. Stickley Co. Philadelphia (in press)

7. Sutow, WW, Wilms' tumor. Methods in Cancer Res 13:31-65, 1976

8. Farber, S, G D'Angio, A Evans, et al, Clinical studies of actinomycin D with special reference to Wilms' tumor in children. Ann NY and Acad Sw 89:421-424, 1960

9. Sutow, WW, WG Thurman and J Windmiller, Vincristine (leurocristine) sulfate in the treatment of children with metastatic Wilms' tumor. Pediatrics 32:880-887, 1963

10. Sullivan, MP and WW Sutow: Successful Therapy for Wilms' Tumor. Texas Med 65:46-51, 1969

11. Sullivan, MP, WW Sutow, A Cangir, et al, Vincristine sulfate in management of Wilms' tumor. Replacement of preoperative irradiation by chemotherapy. JAMA 202:381-384, 1967

12. Bellani, FF, M Gasparini and G Bonadonna, Adriamycin in Wilms' tumor previously treated with chemotherapy. Europ J Cancer 11:593-595, 1975

13. Sutow, WW, Chemotherapy in Wilms tumor, an appraisal. Cancer 32: 1150-1153, 1973

14. D'Angio, GJ, AE Evans, N Breslow, et al, The treatment of Wilms' tumor. Results of the National Wilms' Tumor Study. Cancer 38:633-646, 1976

15. D'Angio, AJ, JB Beckwith, HG Bishop, et al, The National Wilms' Tumor Study: A progress report. Seventh National Cancer Conference Proceedings, J.B. Lippincott Co., Philadelphia/Toronto 1973, p 627-636

242

16. Bishop, HC, M Tefft, AE Evans, et al, Survival in bilateral Wilms' tumor-review of 30 National Wilms' Tumor Study cases. J Pediatr Surg 12:631-638, 1977

17. Beckwith, JB and NF Palmer, Histopathology and prognosis of Wilms' tumor. Cancer 41:1937-1948, 1978

18. National Wilms' Tumor Study Committee: The National Wilms Tumor Study. A report from Cancer Cooperative Study Groups. Cancer Clin Trials 1:61-64, 1978

19. Strong, LC, Genetic and teratogenic aspects of Wilms' tumor. Wilms' Tumor, In Pochedly, C, and Miller, D. (eds), John Wiley & Sons, New York-London-Toronto, 1976, p 63-77

20. Strong, LC, Genetic Consideration in Pediatric Oncology. Clinical Pediatric Oncology (2nd edition), Sutow, WW, TJ Vietti and DJ Fernbach, (eds), C.V. Mosby Co., St. Louis 1977, p 16-327

21. Li, FP, Y Bishop and C Katsioules, Survival in Wilms' tumor. Lancet 1:41-42, 1975

22. Meadows, AT and GJ D'Angio, Late effects of cancer treatment: methods and techniques for detection. Semin Onc 1:87-90, 1974

23. Sutow, WW, Chemotherapeutic management of childhood rhabdomyosarcoma. In: Neoplasia in Childhood, Yearbook Medical Publishers, Chicago, London 1969, p 201-208

24. Donaldson, S, JR Castro, JR Wilbur, et al, Rhabdomyosarcoma of head and neck in children: combination treatment by surgery, irradiation, and chemotherapy. Cancer 31:26-35, 1973

25. Fernandez, CH, WW Sutow, OR Merino, et al, Childhood rhabdomyosarcoma: Analysis of coordinated therapy and results. Am J Roentgenol, Rad Ther Nuc Med 123:588-597, 1975

26. Maurer, HM, The intergroup rhabdomyosarcoma study (NIH): Objectives and clinical staging classification. J Pediatr Surg 10:977-978, 1975

27. Maurer, HM, T Moon, M Donaldson, et al, The intergroup rhabdomyosarcoma study, a preliminary report. Cancer 40:2015-2026, 1977

28. Maurer, HM, M Donaldson, EA Gehan, et al, Rhabdomyosarcoma in childhood and adolescence. Curr Prob Cancer 2:1-36, 1978

29. Maurer, HM, T Moon, M Donaldson, et al, Preliminary results of the Intergroup Rhabdomyosarcoma Study (IRS). Management of Primary Bone and Soft Tissue Tumors. Yearbook Medical Publishers, Chicago, London, 1977, p 317-332

30. Maurer, HM, M Donaldson, EA Gehan, et al, The intergroup rhabdomyosarcoma study - update November, 1978. In Proceedings of Symposium on Sarcoma of Soft Tissue and Bone in Childhood (in press) NCI Monograph

31. Tefft, M, C Fernandez, M Donaldson, et al, Incidence of meningeal involvement by rhabdomyosarcoma of the head and neck in children: A report of the Intergroup Rhabdomyosarcoma Study (IRS). Cancer 42:253-258, 1978

32. Meadows, AT, GJ D'Angio, AE Evans, et al, Oncogenesis and other late effects of cancer treatment in children. Radiology 114:175-180, 1975

33. Intergroup Rhabdomyosarcoma Study Committee: Protocol for IRS-II. (activated Nov., 1978)

34. Marcove, RC, V Mike, JV Hajak, et al, Osteogenic sarcoma under the age of twenty-one. A review of one hundred and forty-five operative cases. J Bone and Joint Surg 52-A:411-423, 1970

35. Sutow, WW, Primary adjuvant chemotherapy in osteosarcoma. Cancer Bull 30:178-181, 1978

36. Sutow, WW, MPM Sullivan, JR Wilbur, et al, Study of adjuvant chemotherapy in osteogenic sarcoma. J Clin Pharm 15:530, 1975

37. Sutow, WW, EA Gehan, TJ Vietti, et al, Multidrug chemotherapy in primary treatment of osteosarcoma. J Bone and Joint Surg 58-A:629-633, 1976

38. Jaffe, N, S Farber, D Traggis, et al, Favorable response of metastatic osteogenic sarcoma to pulse high-dose methotrexate with citrovorum rescue and radiation therapy. Cancer 31:1367-1373, 1973

39. Proceedings of the Osteosarcoma Study Group meeting. Cancer Treat Rep 62:187-312, 1978

40. Gehan, EA. WW Sutow, G Uribe-Botero, et al, Osteosarcoma, In: Immunotherapy of Cancer: Present Status of Trials in Man, The M.D. Anderson Experience, 1950-1974. Terry, WD and D Windhorst, (eds), Raven Press, New York. 1978, p 271-282.

41. Strong, LC, J Herson, BM Osborne, et al, Risk of Radiation-related subsequent malignant tumors in survivors of Ewings' sarcoma. J Nat'l Cancer Inst 62:1401-1406, 1979

AN OVERVIEW OF ADJUVANT THERAPY IN MAN

Emil J Freireich
University of Texas System Cancer Center
M.D. Anderson Hospital and Tumor Institute
Houston, Texas

INTRODUCTION

The concept of "adjuvant therapy" began with the observation that the administration of chemotherapy to patients who have had effective local control of their malignancy with surgery and/or radiation could result in substantial improvement in disease-free interval and survival. Basic to this concept was the idea that these drugs were more effective when administered in association with the primary therapy for local control than when administered only to patients with far advanced disease. This understanding of adjuvant therapy when applied to the role of chemotherapy in the management of patients with malignancy is no longer appropriate, primarily because an "adjuvant" is clearly auxiliary to or enhancing of the benefit of the primary form or forms of treatment. In this role, adjuvant therapy, like antibiotics, nutritional support and other non-specific methods of treatment, is considered as secondary rather than as a major and important component in the overall treatment of the patient's disease. The basic proposition in this paper is that this concept of adjuvant therapy when applied to the use of chemotherapy in patients with early disease should be abandoned and replaced by the concept of multi-modal treatment. In other words, the decision as to whether a given form of therapy is primary or secondary is not crucial. What is crucial is that the choice of the methods of treatment should be appropriate and that the optimal sequence of those methods should be employed to produce an overall strategy for cancer management.

THE MANAGEMENT OF SYSTEMIC CANCER

If cancer were viewed as an illness which always begins in a specific site or specific organ and is derived from a single or small number of cells, then the concept that the aggressive removal of the tumor in its site of origin provides the definitive treatment would appear to be reasonable. Furthermore, if it were accepted that cancers begin in local sites, then spread locally and regionally before they spread to the systemic circulation, then this would strongly support the idea that the early detection and treatment of malignancies with ablative and destructive techniques such as surgery and radiation is a reasonable therapeutic approach, particularly while they are limited to a specific region.

244

This intellectual formulation has led to the strategy of a progressively more radical surgical attack on primary tumors, and progressively more radical radiation therapy approaches, leading ultimately to total body irradiation.

At this phase in our knowledge of the biology of malignant disease in man, we must abandon this old concept of the biology of cancer and recognize the important fact that malignant transformation, even when it occurs in a single cell or a small number of cells, results in the capability of the tumor to extend beyond the normal organ confines of the differentiated stem cells from which it arose. This property of invasiveness is clearly one of the most fundamental changes responsible for the malignant process. Obviously, disorders of proliferation and differentiation which are not associated with the ability to invade give rise to tumors which are benign and totally manageable by local methods such as surgery and radiation. It is, in fact, the property of the cell which allows it to invade, the metastatic potential, which identifies the clinically significant part of the problem (i.e. the cancer) which demands the attention of the clinical scientist and the treating physician. It is clear that tumors have a wide spectrum of ability to invade beyond the site of origin. Therefore, the important undertaking, once the diagnosis of cancer is made, is to assess this metastatic potential and its capability of killing the host. Those tumors which have this metastatic potential as identified by cytologic, histologic or biologic criteria produce a systemic disease and thus local control as primary therapy can only be frustratingly ineffective. Therefore, the diagnostic challenge in cancer treatment is the clear identification of those patients who have systemic disease as opposed to those who have disease which is locally extended and can therefore be managed with primary local therapy. For those patients with systemic malignancy the primary form of therapy must be systemic and the "adjuvant" may or may not include local forms of treatment. For tumors which are confined to local areas, local therapy should be adequate, and adjuvant treatment with systemic therapy is probably harmful to the host and therefore not indicated. Thus, the fundamental change in our perception of malignancy involves identifying those patients who have systemic disease at the time the cancer is recognized and working out the strategy of combined systemic and local therapy which offers the patient the maximum benefit with the least potential risk of toxicity and loss of body organs.

EARLY TREATMENT VS LATE TREATMENT

One of the basic principles in the early development of adjuvant chemotherapy is the important observation that cytotoxic drugs used for systemic chemotherapy have a lethal effect on cells with a dose response that could be described as exponential. In other words, based on repeated in vitro and in vivo observations, for a given exposure to a cytotoxic chemical, the proportion of malignant cells which are killed is relatively constant over a fairly wide range of tumor cell concentrations. Thus, drugs which have only a palliative effect when the number of tumor cells is large, can in fact be curative when the number of tumor cells is small. While this principle has been well documented in cell cultures and in animal tumor models, it depends upon the similarity of tumor growth and the action of the drug upon tumor between those who have clinically detectable disease and those who have micrometastatic disease. There are many clinical observations which indicate that this is probably not the case in human malignancy. One important observation is that certain sites of metastasis have differing susceptibilities to drugs. The pharmacological sanctuary in the central nervous system is a striking example of this, and this phenomenon has been observed not only in the leukemias, but also in a number of other malignancies.

Another important reason that early treatment with chemotherapy is more likely to be effective than later chemotherapy is that the health of the host tissues and organs is significantly better in the patient with early disease than in the patient with advanced disease. Once metastases begin to compromise organ function, the patient's tolerance for systemic therapy is diminished and doses must be compromised. Laboratory and clinical evidence suggests that there is a very steep dose response curve for virtually all of the cancer chemotherapy drugs and that major reductions in effectiveness occur with even minor reductions in dosage or concentration of the drugs. Therefore, the overall performance status of the host, particularly the patient with advanced disease, has proven to be one of the most important prognostic factors in determining the outcome of treatment with chemotherapy.

The potential for more easily tolerating therapy combined with the probability of an improved response because of the smaller volume of malignant tissue, forms an important justification for the earliest use of systemic therapy after the diagnosis of systemic cancer is made, rather than delaying therapy. Chemotherapy thus joins other treatment modalities in being most effectively applied when the least amount of malignant tissue is present. This prompts the therapist to consider chemotherapy in the primary management of the patient rather than reserving it for the advanced stages when it will predictably have only a palliative effect.

HOW TO DIFFERENTIATE SYSTEMIC FROM LOCAL CANCER

The primary responsibility of the physician caring for the patient with cancer is adequate staging of the disease. This staging procedure permits estimation of the probability that the patient has already developed systemic disease. Many important developments have occurred in the field of staging. One example is the use of the carcinoembryonic antigen (CEA) to assist in staging the extent of disease in patients with malignancies of the gastrointestinal tract, the breast, and other organs. Patients who have elevated levels of CEA which return to normal after surgery have a much lower probability of having systemic disease than those in whom the level remains elevated despite what appears to be curative local therapy.

The classic methods for staging the extent of disease revolve primarily around the demonstrated ability of the tumor to invade adjacent tissues. Thus, in melanoma, the thickness and the depth of tumor invasion are clear and strong predictors of the probability of systemic disease. Likewise in breast cancer, the histologic demonstration of malignant cells in regional lymph nodes is a strong indicator that systemic spread of malignancy has already occurred. For each malignancy, depending on its site of origin, there are many factors which independently contribute knowledge about the probability of systemic disease requiring systemic therapy. Many of these factors, of course, are interrelated. For instance, the size of a breast primary is correlated with the probability of lymph node involvement. Likewise, cytologic grade of malignancy in the primary is also correlated with regional spread. Therefore, it is important to develop methods for analyzing such multiple interrelated factors simultaneously in order to reach quantitative estimates of the likelihood of systemic disease at the time of diagnosis. Multifactorial statistical analyses are thus being used increasingly to assess the probability of systemic disease. The application of these statistical methods allows for the identification of those patients with a high probability of systemic disease who would most likely benefit, and possibly be cured, by the early application of systemic therapy.

WHICH MODALITY OF CANCER TREATMENT IS THE "ADJUVANT"?

Once the diagnostic staging procedure is completed, if the patient has a high probability of systemic disease, it becomes clear that the primary treatment modality is to be systemic therapy or chemotherapy. Any indicated local forms of therapy, such as surgery or irradiation, would then be adjuvant to the primary treatment. At the other extreme, of course, patients who have a low probability of systemic disease should have local therapy as their primary treatment modality and chemotherapy must be considered adjuvant. The question as to which treatment modality is primary is of more than minor importance, because systemic disease will progress unabated during the time devoted to local control in patients who receive only local therapy initially. For both surgery and irradiation, this may involve months of therapy or recovery from therapy and this time may be significant in the natural history of the disease. Potentially curable systemic illness (micrometastases) may become incurable while the local therapy is being administered. Therefore, the choice of the primary treatment modality affects the overall therapeutic strategy for such patients. The proper sequence of treatment therefore depends to a great extent upon the diagnostic staging evaluation of each patient with malignancy, and an assessment of the probability of systemic disease.

Perhaps more importantly, the decision as to which treatment is adjuvant also raises the question: "Who is the doctor?" With our present methods of cancer diagnosis and staging, it is essential to obtain a portion of the tumor by a surgical procedure, and therefore the surgical specialist is frequently the original physician involved in outlining the overall treatment strategy. In many centers and institutions, it has become the practice for surgeons to actually supervise the systemic therapy or the chemotherapy. This is no more logical than to ask the medical oncologist who specializes in chemotherapy to be responsible for the surgical modality of treatment, or for the radiotherapy. If systemic treatment, or chemotherapy, is to be considered in the primary management of the patient, then the medical oncologist must be involved in the original treatment decisions in order to assure that it be included if indicated and, perhaps more importantly, that it be administered in the most technically efficient dose and sequence. This is the field of expertise of the medical oncologist.

For many malignancies, technically efficient and effective local therapy is a significant part of the staging of the patient's disease. For example, in melanoma, resection of adequate tissue to assess the level of invasion is crucial in consideration of prognosis. Likewise, in breast cancer, evaluation of regional lymph node involvement is an important phase of determining the extent of disease. Therefore, the local surgical management frequently takes sequential precedence because it is involved in the staging procedure. However, as improvements are achieved in regional control with radiation therapy and systemic control with chemotherapy, modifications in the surgical strategy are being made. For example, at many centers, in the staging of breast cancer axillary lymph nodes are now only biopsied rather than removed in contiguity.

Thus, the proper sequence for modalities of treatment is currently evolving in an effort to preserve the original organ function in its most advantageous form.

THE REQUIREMENTS FOR INCLUSION OF CHEMOTHERAPY
IN THE MULTIMODAL MANAGEMENT OF MALIGNANCY[1-4]

Drugs in those schedules which result in substantial regression of advanced disease have been identified as useful, and should be used also for early treatment of malignancy. Conversely, drugs or schedules which have unknown, minimal or no effectiveness against advanced disease should not be used for early treatment. When ineffective drugs have been used in adjuvant chemotherapy studies, they have resulted in minimal or marginal benefits to the patients, and have generally produced toxicity. It seems quite fruitless in the adjuvant setting to employ drugs in dosages or schedules which are known to be without effect in advanced disease. There have been sufficient studies to demonstrate that such strategies will not be effective. For example, in the case of colon cancer, the literature is extremely confusing. This is because chemotherapy for advanced metastatic colon cancer is, at best, only minimally effective with less than half of the patients showing any objective regression, and these treatments have to be given in doses which have considerable toxicity for the host. Thus, the literature on the use of chemotherapy adjuvant to surgery for colon cancer is full of falsely negative studies where inadequate doses of a marginally effective drug are being evaluated. It is not surprising that the outcomes reveal no effective benefit to the patient. In breast cancer, on the other hand, individual drugs and combinations of drugs have shown objective response in a large percentage of patients with metastatic disease and it is now clear that chemotherapy given as adjuvant to surgery is effective in prolonging the disease free interval and survival. Thus, it is clear that the choice of treatment for patients with early cancer must be drawn from treatments of proven value for patients with advanced disease.

The quantitative assessment of effectiveness of treatment in advanced disease is particularly important in this connection. It is now clear that drugs which produce partial objective regressions of 50% or more in advanced disease are not sufficient to have detectable effects on early disease except in tumors that have extremely long doubling times. When chemotherapy for advanced disease results in detectable frequencies of complete remission, then the use of these drugs in patients with early disease is strongly indicated and to date has consistently given beneficial outcomes for the patients so treated. Thus, evaluation of chemotherapy regimens as adjuvant to local control requires that complete remissions (that is, more than 90% regressions) be observed in a detectable fraction of patients with the advanced metastatic form of that disease. Such treatment regimens are attractive as adjuvant therapy.

ADJUVANT THERAPY LESSONS
FROM THE TREATMENT OF ACUTE LEUKEMIA

Adult acute leukemia is a disease which is almost uniformly systemic at the time it is diagnosed. Because it arises from the stem cells of the bone marrow, an organ which is widely dispersed throughout the flat bones of the body, the tumor cells have ready access to the blood and metastasize very early in the evolution of this disease. Thus it is rarely, if ever, diagnosed while confined to a local or regional area. This form of systemic cancer, therefore, serves as an important prototype for the development of ideas relating to adjuvant therapy.

Until recently objective complete remissions (greater than 90% reduction in the amount of leukemic disease associated with complete recovery of the myeloid bone marrow function and restoration of normal concentrations of formed elements in the peripheral blood) were observed in less than 10% of the treated patients with acute leukemia. Stated negatively, 90% of patients with this diagnosis showed only minor regressions of tumor with available drugs. At the present time, more than 2/3 of patients with acute leukemia can be restored to a clinical condition indistinguishable from normal with combination chemotherapy regimens. Thus, 2/3 of patients today with a documented form of systemic far advanced "stage IV" malignancy can be restored to a condition in which they have no evidence of residual disease. It then becomes necessary to identify the reasons for failure to induce remission in the 1/3 of patients with this tumor who fail to respond, in order to modify chemotherapy for these patients in the hope of achieving long-term remissions or cures. Multifactorial statistical techniques, (especially stepwise forward regression analysis) using currently available combination therapy, does in fact identify a group of patients who have a poor probability of responding.[5] The factors which help to predict the probability of response include the age at the time of diagnosis (with youth as a favorable factor), no history of pre-leukemic bone marrow disturbance preceding the onset of leukemia, and the morphological diagnosis of disease (that is, myeloblastic or differentiated acute leukemia versus lymphoblastic or undifferentiated leukemia).[6] Creation of a logistic regression equation as a model for predicting probability of response allows the calculation of the exact probability of response to primary treatment for each patient. Thus, patient populations with over 80% probability of response can be identified which are certainly candidates for administration of currently available combination chemotherapy. In contrast, one can also identify patients with a very low probability of response to the existing treatments, and it would seem futile to treat these patients with current treatments. It is for this poor prognosis group that new systemic therapy is needed and justified in order to improve the probability of response.

If treatment is administered until the patient is free of disease and then discontinued, the disease will recur promptly in virtually all of the patients without further treatment. The median time to relapse is two to three months and more than 90% recur within 8 months. Thus, with our current methods for estimating residual leukemic disease, it is clear that the patient in complete remission, while rendered free of objective evidence of disease, still has residual systemic leukemia which will recur in the absence of further treatment. Thus, for acute leukemia, the process of remission induction is analogous to the process of primary local treatment for the solid tumors. For example, a post-mastectomy breast cancer patient whose staging revealed more than four involved axillary lymph nodes or unfavorable local signs in the breast is in a high-risk category for recurrence. That patient is in a situation similar to the patient with leukemia in complete remission, in that there is micrometastatic disease with a high probability of recurrence.

Now that a high percentage of complete remissions can be attained, the important consideration is the choice of treatment (i.e. adjuvant therapy) for the patient in remission in contrast to the patient with extensive disease. In acute leukemia, we have recently documented that the factors which predict for duration of the disease free interval or duration of remission are entirely different from those factors which predict for probability of remission.[7] One factor affecting response duration is sensitivity to drugs. Thus, the prognosis of the patient in complete resmision is affected by the sensitivity of the disease to the treatment chosen as adjuvant. In leukemia, this can be assessed by the rapidity of regression of the documented disease in the blood and bone marrow. The recent introduction of in vitro techniques for evaluating drug sensitivity of the cells offers the prospect of applying the same principle to a number of solid tumors as well. The second group of factors influencing the duration of the disease free interval or the duration of remission relates to the extent of disease prior to the onset of remission induction therapy. Thus, patients with greatly elevated serum lactate dehydrogenase levels or extensive invasion of the blood have a higher probability of relapse even though they achieve the same quality of complete response. This, of course, is strongly analogous to the solid tumor situation in which the extent of both the primary and local invasion are the most significant factors predicting for probability of systemic relapse. Thus, in leukemia, a systemic disease at the outset, the choice of combination chemotherapy for local control renders the patient free of disease and accomplishes both staging and debulking objectives. In other words, it reduces the body burden of tumor and restores organ function to as nearly normal as possible.

In the adjuvant situation, the patient has no objective evidence of residual disease, and we are therefore attempting to devise a treatment which will eliminate micrometastatic disease and result in prolongation of the disease free interval. This is an enormous challenge for the clinical scientist since it involves the decision to render potentially toxic treatment in the absence of objective evidence of disease and in the presence of a finite but detectable probability that the patient is already cured by the local treatment. In leukemia there is evidence that a small fraction of patients is, in fact, disease free with minimum treatment. With continued chemotherapy during remission, it can be demonstrated that at least 15 to 25 percent of patients who receive effective treatment for more than one year following the induction of remission have prolonged disease free periods in excess of two to three years. Patients who remain disease free for that period of time have a greatly diminished risk of recurrence. Thus, the choice of treatment for the patient who has no evidence of disease must be based on quantitative and objective evaluation of the risk of recurrence. The choice of adjuvant therapy must be influenced by documented improvements in disease free interval and decrease in relapse in the patient populations studied.

TREATMENT OF THE PATIENT
WHO HAS NO EVIDENCE OF RESIDUAL DISEASE

The concept of adjuvant treatment should be replaced with the concept of therapy given to patients who have no clinical evidence of residual cancer. This is the prototype for the adjuvant situation. If a patient with systemic metastatic cancer has complete remission and therefore no evidence of disease, does local therapy either to the primary site or to sites of massive disease improve the overall salvage rate or the quality of the palliative effect as measured by prolongation of disease free interval? This question is under active investigation by many investigators. Likewise, in the surgically treated patient, is radiation therapy indicated for extended local control? Can it be justified, considering increased morbidity? Even more difficult, however, are the decisions involving the use of chemotherapy where morbidity is frequently high compared to the other modalities of treatment.

The primary problem in the treatment of the patient without residual disease is objective, accurate, quantitative and expert evaluation of benefit/risk ratios. This is a term widely used and abused in the lay literature, but a concept which clinical scientists cannot avoid. For each patient, the potential for benefit by early treatment in the absence of clinical disease must be balanced with all of the morbidity, cost, inconvenience, etc., associated with the administration of treatment. The decision-making process of the clinician should begin with the development of objective, quantitative criteria and the use of multifactorial statistical techniques for converting multiple factors into single quantitative statements of risk. This requires extensive knowledge, analysis and understanding of our historical data in order to prescribe therapy, and also to guide clinical trials in adjuvant treatment. Knowledge of the patients at high risk of relapse would induce highly developmental treatment programs to be used in such patient populations. In contrast, where a low risk of recurrence exists, it seems clear that observation of the patient for the earliest detectable evidence of either residual or recurrent disease along with treatment for remission induction is the wiser strategy.

SUMMARY

Now that chemotherapy can be curative in a small but detectable fraction of patients with demonstrated metastatic disease, it must be considered for possible treatment of patients with early disease. The major questions to be resolved in cancer management are: 1) the intelligent choice of modalities of treatment which are necessary and sufficient for controlling any malignancy; 2) whether multiple modes of treatment are indicated; and 3) the choice of treatment strategy (the sequence of treatments). Increasingly, chemotherapy is assuming the role of primary treatment for patients with malignancy with surgery and radiation therapy serving as adjuvants. While a growing number of early stage solid tumors are being adequately managed with surgery and radiation, chemotherapy has proven effective in advanced disease and is being used as adjuvant to local control. Because this "multi-modal" strategy offers a wide range of therapeutic options, the knowledge and expertise of the practitioners of each modality of treatment must be involved in treatment planning for a growing number of patients with malignant disease. For each patient with malignancy, the primary requirement is for adequate staging to assess the possibility of his having systemic disease at the time of diagnosis. Based upon that knowledge, the secondmost important question is whether the benefit/risk ratios support the recommendation for treatment of a patient who has no objective evidence of residual disease, but has the risk of systemic disease.

REFERENCES

1. Buzdar, AU, JU Gutterman, GR Blumenschein, et al, Intensive postoperative chemoimmunotherapy for patients with stage II and stage III breast cancer. Ca 41:1064-1075, 1978

2. Mavligit, GM, JU Gutterman, MA Malahy, et al, Adjuvant immunotherapy and chemoimmunotherapy for colorectal cancer (Duke's Class C). Cancer 40:2726-2730, 1977

3. Proceedings of the Osteosarcoma Study Group Meeting (Bethesda, Maryland, January, 1977). Cancer Treat Rep 62:187-313, 1978

4. Gutterman, JU, GM Mavligit, SP Richman, et al, Adjuvant immunotherapy of melanoma, an updated report. Proceedings of the 22nd Annual M.D. Anderson Clinical Conference, November, 1977. Immunotherapy of Human Cancer (in press)

5. Freireich EJ, MJ Keating, EA Gehan, et al, Therapy of acute myelogenous leukemia. Cancer 42:874-882, 1978

6. Gehan, EA, TL Smith, EJ Freireich, et al, Prognostic factors in acute leukemia. Semin Onc 3:271-282, 1976

7. Keating, MJ, TL Smith, EA Gehan, et al, Factors related to length of complete remission in adult acute leukemia. Cancer (in press)

AN OVERVIEW OF UNCONVENTIONAL (FRAUDULENT) TREATMENTS OF CANCER

Daniel S. Martin

Catholic Medical Center

New York, New York

INTRODUCTION

Cancer fear runs rampant, and it is not polite to even question the so-called facts. Frequent news stories, television documentaries and magazine features often refer to an "epidemic" of cancer as the price for the benefits of modern civilization. Today everyone seems to believe that the additives, synthetic colorings, flavorings and hormones in food, the water we drink, the polluted air we breathe, cigarettes, hair dyes, saccharine, cyclamates, etc. etc. - you name it - everything is suspected, proven, or feared as a cancer-causing agent, a carcinogen. And so it is popular to believe that modern technology has made us victims of adulterated, over-processed food, and filled our workplaces and total environment with cancer-causing chemicals.

Contrary to media assertions, there is no general cancer epidemic. When population increase and age-adjustment are taken into account, and cancers of the respiratory tract are removed from consideration, the overall cancer incidence is found to have decreased slightly since 1950. The recent increase in cancer incidence is limited entirely to lung cancer. However, it is not germane to this article to discuss this facet of the cancer problem. Cancer - apparently considered the most frightening disease of all - in the trade parlance of the media, "sells". Thus, media hype has led to ever-increasing public acceptance that there is a cancer epidemic, and aroused public concern about what to do about it (e.g., prevention research vs. treatment research). Today, cancer has become a shrill political issue.

NUTRITION AND CANCER

In the uncertainty and confusion concerning the cause(s) of cancer, nutrition is often cited as a possible environmental factor, and the nutritional quacksters are having a "field day". To understand this phenomenon it should be recognized that food has always had a role in medicine and folk tradition. Through the ages food has been of central importance to man. Major religions have concerned themselves with food. Witness the Biblical injunction of the Jews against pork, or the religious vegetarian food practices of the Hindus. There has always been a vast food folklore, such as the belief that garlic possesses a mystic healing

256

potency. There is the simplistic notion that "we are what we eat", and children are admonished to eat food that is "good for you" and to avoid food that is "bad for you". The allure of food fads, and food cults has complex and deep-reaching roots. There are many false beliefs about food, and fake food cures for chronic disease problems are a major public health problem in America. The public is deceived by individuals who exaggerate facts and deal in pseudoscience.

The problem is complicated in that the nutritional appeal is inadvertently helped along by science. There is, of course, validity to the study of nutrition and cancer. Hence, there are proper scientific reports in the literature about dietary links to cancer. Cancer often induces loss of appetite with accompanying severe weight loss and drastic deterioration of the patient. It is not surprising that improving the cancer patient's nutrition has been shown by medical scientists to enhance the patient's immunologic status, as well as the ability to better tolerate cancer treatments such as chemotherapy. Such scientific studies frequently are reported in the public media. Twisted by the quacks to their purpose, these reports lend a respectable background to their misleading discussions about nutrition and cancer.

I recently received a somewhat amusing letter from a stranger, a layperson, who explained these matters in the following way: "I assume you are aware that ... (fake cancer treatments are being advanced) ... by an 'underground' of medical doctors who call themselves 'nutritionists'." Now, I am familar with some of their theories and they are just near enough to the truth to be convincing. But, since to talk intelligently about any subject requires almost as much expertise as the professional, they are able to fool many people on crucial points. They are not quacks or fakers - if they were they could be dealt with. They are fanatics. They are sure - but absolutely sure - they are right. And there is no doubt that for many people changes in diet are beneficial, not because nutritionist theories of disease and malfunction are valid, but because most people are eating unadulterated crap - you will pardon the expression. Thus, you have a deadly situation - fanatics, with theories that are not really that erroneous, provided they do not define disease in nutritional terms, and the fact that some of the courses of behavior they recommend are "beneficial".

NUTRITIONAL MISINFORMATION

Through books, pamphlets, mail-order advertising, radio and television, "health" conventions, sales conversations in "health food" stores, media articles, and special "health" magazines, cancerophobia is promoted. The books are very well-written, with clever subtleties and innuendoes that are misleading, with exaggerated facts boldly interspersed with blatant untruths, and with references to erroneous research. Our freedom of speech laws protect the quack - anybody can write or preach any false health statement. The FDA can only act against misleading labels on products.

Quack pseudonutritional medicine promotes its cause by spreading misinformation about health and nutrition, and by undermining faith in the regular food supply. The promotors are also clever at turning real facts to their advantage. For example, they cunningly over-emphasize a possible cancer risk in food additive, but do not reveal that its cancer-causing potential is only an assumption; that is, a scientifically hypothetical risk. Of 120 pesticides thought to be possible carcinogens only 11 have been shown to be cancer-causing, and then only in animals. Nevertheless, they will take advantage of these facts, cunningly extrapolate from the assumptions, and inflame further the highly emotionally-charged fear of cancer.

Nutrition seems to be a subject that all feel they can understand. Everyone is either knowledgeable, claims to be, or feels that, without any background, he can nevertheless learn all he or she needs by reading any so-called nutritional publication. The field of nutrition is filled with dogmatic statements, some of which are true, some of which are false, and many of which are still to be determined. The so-called "facts" that are being stated frequently have nothing to do with what is scientifically proven about metabolic pathways, cell and organ physiology, or even common sense. No matter, for the uninformed, the ignorant and the faithful, believing is all that matters. In the cancer area, desperation, the fear of becoming one of the desperately ill, and wishful thinking apparently wipe out all reason. Thus, there are many so-called "nutrition experts" who broadcast nutritional misinformation on radio programs, on TV talk shows, and in "health" books, although they have had virtually no nutritional or health science training. Despite this, their articles are sought by "health" publications that are replete with nutritional misinformation. The reasons for all this activity are simple. There is "big money" to be made in food quackery; and, as stated earlier, anybody can write or preach any false health statement without fear of legal reprisal.

WHY ARE PEOPLE SO VULNERABLE TO EXPLOITATION
IN THE FIELD OF NUTRITION?

There is widespread belief that the food industry has overpurified processed foods, that certain key nutritional elements (such as vitamins) have been removed, that the so-called "naturalness" of the food is gone. An example of the attempt to manipulate the public in this regard is the claim that "organically-grown food" is grown differently from "regular" food - this is true - and therefore is nutritionally superior to "regular" food - this is untrue. Chemicals, whether provided by artificial or "natural" (manure) fertilizers, are all utilized by plants in their inorganic natural state. No differences have been found in major nutrient values between organically grown and regular foods. Nor should there be. After all, nutritional factors in food are controlled by the plant's genes. Yet, the organic food lobby utilizes publications to spread misleading "health" information to frighten the public into buying their product. They profit greatly because food labeled "organic" usually has a very large mark-up. To claim that organic food is qualitatively superior to regular food is false scare propaganda for personal profit.

The nutritional quacks vigorously lobby congress for the "freedom to choose" unproven cancer remedies. It is not surprising for politicians to develop personal biases in favor of pressure groups who furnish campaign funds, or who promise blocs of votes. The quacks are well-organized, well-financed, and cunning. For example, their "freedom of choice" policy states that they "oppose the efforts of any one group to restrict the freedom of practice of qualified members of another profession". Behind these piously stated words with the good old-fashioned ring of Americanism lurks their real goal: the true facts (i.e., science) should not be allowed to drive quackery out of the marketplace.

THE "FREEDOM OF CHOICE" ARGUMENT IS
A CONSUMER PROTECTION TRAP

The "freedom of choice" argument was commented upon in published hearings by the U.S. Senate's Subcommittee on Health and Scientific Resources (July 12, 1977) as follows: "The elimination of useless treatment is a valid Federal role. It is a humanitarian role. It reduces the burden on cancer patients and their families and allows them to exercise their freedom of choice on the basis of informed judgments among viable alternatives".

The key word is "informed". The chooser must be properly informed, which is to say that the imparted information must be true, a "viable" alternative. The patient and family do not want to consider hearsay remedies - they seek a reliable treatment that may lead to cure. "Freedom of choice" requires that the patient be informed truthfully as to the real alternative choices.

Certainly, "freedom of choice" should not include the freedom to defraud. The seller's desire to make money should not condone the license to misrepresent facts. Caveat emptor - "let the buyer beware" - is an immoral, unethical and particularly reprehensible doctrine in the medical marketplace where human life is at stake. Thus, the FDA has been given statutory authority by the people to allow only drugs to reach the marketplace that are proven efficacious and safe. The "freedom of choice" argument, slyly wrapped in an American flag, is merely specious logic contrived to destroy consumer protection. Only the unscrupulous can benefit. Under such "freedom of choice" the uninformed, the naive, the innocent, the fanatics, the very poor, the very young, and the very desperately sick, will buy a fraud from the unscrupulous, thinking it a treatment.

The "Nuremberg Code" was formulated as a guide to protect human subjects. One of its principles is applicable: "...the person involved ... should be able to exercise free power of choice, without the intervention of any element of force, fraud, deceit, duress, over-reaching, or any other ulterior form of constraint or coercion ... The ... (treatment) ... should be based on the results of animal experimentation and a knowledge of the natural history of the disease ... (so) ... that the anticipated results (will) justify the performance of the ... (treatment) ..."

THE UNSCRUPULOUS AND THE MISGUIDED PHYSICIAN

There are, of course, unscrupulous individuals, and medicine is not immune. There are also misguided, or uninformed and unscholarly physicians, who simply do not know that in its natural progression, cancer may frequently show stable periods, rather than inexorable growth leading quickly to death. Cancer is a chronic disease; some people with advanced cancer can live for years before succumbing. If an inexperienced physician naively treated a cancer patient with a fraudulent remedy before a stable period, the unknowing physician might conclude erroneously that the treatment was effective. No physician is well-trained in everything. There are many physicians with little training and experience in oncology, who have a small knowledge of recent advances in the field. A problem for the layman, then, is to recognize the genuine authority and expert in the field of cancer. But this problem is really inconsiderable. An expert in any particular field is an individual qualified by recognized scientific training and experience in that field. There are published data available in any good library that will provide such information. As for the unscrupulous expert, he can be perceived simply by his opinion being not "generally" recognized by most qualified experts in the field. To insist on viewing either unknowing or charlatan physicians as brave, independently-minded "pioneers" is naive, wishful thinking, and represents the mindless conquest of false hope over the facts.

THE TESTIMONIAL, THE ANECDOTE, AND THE PLACEBO EFFECT

An understanding of the "placebo effect" is central to understanding the success of quack cancer cures. A placebo is an inactive preparation for the disease being treated, but which is psychologically effective due to the power of suggestion attendant upon its administration. Emotions have a strong effect on a patient's perception of being helped by a medicine. If a frightened ill patient is led to believe that his hopes are being met with the promise of cure due to the administration of what in reality is a placebo, his despair can be transiently relieved and attendant euphoria can temporarily overcome feelings of pain and malaise. Many studies have shown that 30% to 40% of patients with post-operative pain can be relieved by sugar pills and injections of water -- namely, placebos. This unreal but patient-perceived effectiveness of a drug - the "placebo effect" - is well-recognized in the field of medicine. The self-deluded patient derives the psychological benefit of feeling better and on his way to recovery.

Cancer is a chronic disease with a natural history of intermittent periods of "ups" and "downs". It is therefore not hard to understand how a cancer victim might be lead to believe that he is benefitting from a quack "cure". To begin with, a feeling of benefit is experienced due to the "placebo effect". Subsequently, this feeling can be fortified by an "up" occasioned in the natural course of the disease. The result is a testimonial by the patient, and a supporting anecdote by observers.

These claims may be quite sincere, but the "placebo effect" is all too often the obvious explanation. This is evidenced by findings that some of those who believe themselves cured of cancer by a quack cure were erroneously (or falsely) diagnosed; they simply never had cancer. Others, who did have documented cancer, were not objectively effected by the "cure"; indeed, subsequent to their testimonials regarding the efficacy of the "cure", they died of the disease. And still others received concurrent proven effective therapies (e.g., surgery, or radiotherapy, or chemotherapy) which appear to have produced the actual benefit, although the patient ascribes the benefit solely to the quack "cure". No matter how sincere, the testimonial is subjective, and cannot substitute for objective scientific data.

THE "TERMINAL" ARGUMENT

The placebo effect that can accompany the administration of any drug, including quack drugs, has been advanced by proponents of the latter as reason enough to allow "terminal" cancer patients to have such bogus treatment. Their justification is that, since such patients are beyond the help of proven therapies, the quack "cure" cannot hurt and the patient will derive psychological benefit. This argument recently has been declared invalid by the Supreme Court. The Court unanimously declared that the Food and Drug Act's "safe and effective" standard protects both the terminally ill as well as patients suffering curable diseases. Thus, all patients are entitled to equal protection in that drugs must be shown safe and effective before marketing.

Regardless of this logical and gratifying legal ruling, the "terminally ill" prognosis angle is also medically invalid. No physician can predict accurately either the survival time of an individual patient, or which patients surely will die of their disease. Prognostic statements are based on genereal results in which the individual's "fit" into the overall statistics can only be "guesstimated". Also, prognostic statements are based on past results, and newer drug treatments are continuously changing these past statistics. A small but growing fraction of so-called "terminal" cancer patients now have long disease-free periods, and some are even cured, by participating in new clinical research programs.

Since there is no way of knowing which patients have reached the dying phase of their disease until after the fact of death, the taking of quack "cures" diverts some patients from truly promising therapies that might in fact cure some of them. The phrase "terminal" prognosis should be abandoned for the more accurate terminology of "grim" prognosis. The former term implies certainty of fatal outcome and such accuracy is not possible, whereas the latter term allows the possibility that some patients may overcome their disease. The latter is prognostically correct, and compassionately offers real hope as opposed to the false hopes of the medical quacks.

Granting a person who is presumed under a cancer death sentence his or her "last" wishes may seem innocent and virtuous. Such compassion is ill-conceived in the light of the higher moral imperative of the general welfare. People will be lead to believe that the placebo must have an anticancer effect if all - especially the physician - conspire to such false presentation. Governmental (legal) approval of such a drug will lend credibility to such illusion. This is a dangerous deception, for the unscrupulous will then spread propaganda that, if the placebo "helps" the "terminally ill", then it will "work" better on early cancer, and also as a preventive before one gets cancer. This line of reasoning can (and does) lure people into taking unconventional (fraudulent) treatments in preference to proven medical therapy. The harm in taking the quack "cure" is that precious time is lost while cancer advances to the point where no cure by conventional treatment is possible. Compassion for a gravely ill person's desperately conceived "last wishes" cannot be allowed to take precedence over the larger issue of concern for the public welfare. "Helping" a relatively few dying advanced cancer patients, while luring a far larger number of early (potentially curable) cancer patients to a "point of no return", is not an acceptable trade-off. The overall gain in public protection substantially outweighs the option of compassion for the few. Indeed, on many issues the overall public interest overrides the right of freedom of choice for the individual in our society. And, in final analysis, the "terminally ill" argument is just the "freedom of choice" argument in another guise.

THE UNCONVENTIONAL (FRAUDULENT) TREATMENTS FOR CANCER

Quackery has always been successful in the cancer field. The main reason is fear. Cancer engenders fear. Even the hope that proven therapies for cancer offers is often offset by the reason that the legitimate therapies themselves (e.g., surgery as in a mastectomy, or the toxic side-effects of chemotherapy) give rise to fear. Place alongside these facts the testimonials that "it works and isn't toxic" and that there are many who are naive or unknowing and distrustful of government and the medical establishment, and the setting is ripe for exploitation by the unscrupulous. Thus, through the years, cancerophobia has engendered acceptance of claims that special unconventional treatment will either control, or cure, or prevent cancer.

Throughout the ages there have been hundreds and hundreds of supposed remedies. To name only a few in modern times, there is the Zen Macrobiotic Diet, the "Grape Cure", the Chase Dietary Method, "Koch Antitoxins", the Hoxsey Method, Krebiozen, the Rand Vaccine, the Bahamas "Immunologic" Treatment and Laetrile with special diets that include the mystic use of daily coffee enemas. For many, fear propels acceptance of the outlandish and the unreasonable.

LAETRILE

The most "successful" of all forms of cancer quackery is Laetrile. Laetrile (or amygdalin), a compound derived primarily from apricot pits, has been branded worthless as a cancer treatment by every major establishment in the United States, including state medical societies, the American Medical Association, the Committee on Neoplastic Diseases of the American Academy of Pediatrics, the American Cancer Society, the American Society of Clinical Oncology, the National Cancer Institute, key cancer research organizations (e.g., the Memorial Sloan-Kettering Cancer Institute) and the Food and Drug Administration.

Laetrile has been heralded by its promotors as the anticancer "vitamin", but recognized nutritional authorities in the United States have termed this false propaganda. Laetrile is neither a vitamin, nor an anticancer agent.

The Supreme Court has unanimously upheld the Federal government's authority to ban importation and transportation of Laetrile as illegal in interstate commerce because the FDA has found Laetrile not proven to be safe and efficacious. The drug has been termed toxic and dangerous, and deaths have been reported in both the lay and medical press.

It has been widely publicized that the principal promotors of Laetrile do not have the appropriate credentials in research or medical or oncological competence. Some have criminal records or have convictions for practicing medicine without a license, or, if M.D.'s, have had their M.D. license removed for incompetence. And, all have made huge fortunes from the sale of Laetrile.

Despite all of the obviously negative "caveat emptor" information available to the public on this quack drug, Laetrile's advocates have persuaded seventeen states to adopt laws legalizing its manufacture and sale within the state. A widespread black market in Laetrile smuggled into the United States from Mexico, Europe and South America exists. It is estimated that 50,000 to 75,000 Americans take it regularly, and their numbers are believed to be growing.

WHY DO PEOPLE PLACE THEIR LIVES, OR THE LIVES OF THEIR LOVED ONES ON A TREATMENT WHICH IS GENERALLY REJECTED AS A FRAUD BY ALMOST EVERYONE TRAINED AND EXPERIENCED IN CANCER RESEARCH AND TREATMENT?

A number of the answers to this question have already been given or implied - unreasoning fear of cancer, a belief in nutrition and vitamins as a panacea for disease, hostility to scientific medicine, antagonism to government authority, right wing politics, an inability to separate anecdote from scientific fact, religious fundamentalism, gullibility as evidenced by an inadequacy or unwilling-ness to differentiate between pseudo-scientific "experts" and legitimate scientific authorities on nutrition and cancer, a willingness by state legislators to seek votes without respect to the obligation to seek truth, incapacity to perceive the inappropriateness of the specious "freedom of choice" and "terminal cancer" arguments, and skillful use of the mass media including books, popular journalism, cult publications, radio and television, and word of mouth through organized meetings and conventions.

HOW UNCONVENTIONAL (FRAUDULENT) TREATMENTS OF CANCER ARE SUCCESSFULLY PROMOTED - HOW LAYPEOPLE ARE DECEIVED - LAETRILE AS AN EXAMPLE

All unconventional (fraudulent) treatments of cancer have been similarly promoted. Laetrile is a typical example of the usual historical pattern of other unproven cancer remedies. A review of Laetrile is therefore presented, since comprehension of one such fraud facilitates an understanding of them all. Moreover, and importantly, such knowledge will enable earlier perception of the next fraud. It must be recognized that as long as cancer remains an unsolved problem, and the unscrupulous and the gullible reside amongst us, there will be a "next" fraudulent cancer remedy.

The headings below indicate the similarities in manner of promotion of supposed cancer remedies, while the more detailed paragraph discussions reveal how Laetrile's promotion was actually done.

"Scientific" Claims without Supporting Data

The proponents don the mantle of scientific terminology. The Laetrile theory proposes that a component of Laetrile, hydrogen cyanide, is released in cancer cells because they contain the enzyme beta-glucosidase, while normal cells are protected because they contain another enzyme (rhodonase) which detoxifies cyanide. Despite findings that there are no such enzymatic differences between normal and cancerous tissue, the Laetrilists nevertheless continue to make these false assertions.

The Laetrilists also claim that laboratory studies evidenced therapeutic activity by Laetrile against animal cancer. In contrast, all animal studies by researchers generally recognized as competent in the cancer field were reported negative (except for one early study which was not subsequently confirmed, even when repeated by the original scientist of record).

Testimonials for Clinical Evidence

The Laetrilists present case histories to support their claim that Laetrile has clinical benefits. However, these claims have turned out to be hearsay or subjective evidence (i.e., anecdotes and testimonials). Their claims for pain relief fall only into the range expected for a "placebo effect". There is no objective data.

In Hoxsey's day of quackery, he claimed he could not "spare the time, personnel, and facilities for objective study" because he was too busy treating cancer patients. Nothing has changed. Today's physician-advocate of Laetrile,

Dr. E. Contreras, states "We have neither the time nor the personnel to be a research institute. We are too busy treating patients".

Claim is Made That Cancer Causation Is Due To Diet

As is common to other unproven cancer remedies, the claim is that cancer is a nutritional deficiency disease, and the Laetrile is the missing anti-cancer vitamin B_{17}. No evidence is presented that cancer is a nutritional deficiency disease, or that Laetrile is a vitamin. They ignore the findings of recognized nutritional experts that there is no such vitamin as B_{17}.

Claim of Non-Toxicity

Laetrile, like all other unproven cancer remedies, is promoted as a harmless cancer remedy free of the side-affects associated with orthodox methods of treatment such as surgery, radiation, and chemotherapy. Yet, the facts are documented that some patients taking Laetrile have died from the cyanide in Laetrile.

Moreover, even if the drug were harmless (which it obviously is not), there is no evidence that it is efficacious. A useful drug should not merely be non-toxic, but it should beneficially effect the disease process (and not just the promoter's bank account).

Claim for Equality of Opinion

The Laetrilists do not require that an expert be qualified by scientific training and experience to evaluate the safety and effectiveness of drugs. Any opinion supportive of Laetrile, regardless of the individual's lack of background as scientist or oncologist, is, they feel, to be accorded equal weight with that of experts recognized according to the above-defined criteria.

Yet key promoters of Laetrile have backgrounds as follows: One has been convicted for stock fraud and other brushes with the law; one poses as an engineer but never received the degree; one has posed as a physician but has not the degree; one is a physician but has had his M.D. degree removed for malpractice; one has only a college degree but poses as a biochemist and has the gall to proclaim a substance as a vitamin; one is a board-trained psychiatrist but claims he is nevertheless a cancer expert although he has no background of training in oncology.

Claim Persecution As Scientific Pioneers

It is noteworthy that quacks never refer to "scientific" medicine as their opposition, for that might lead to the quack's characterization as "unscientific". Rather, they refer to "orthodox" or "conventional" medicine, so they can term themselves "unorthodox" or "unconventional", and thereby imply heroic, creative scientific originality. For example, Laetrilists compare their "pioneers" with earlier scientists such as Copernicus, Newton, Freud, Galileo, and Semmelweiss, who were persecuted for their now accepted theories.

Claim "Establishment" Prejudice and a Conspiracy

The proponents of Laetrile have often accused governmental agencies and organized medicine of a "cover-up" to hide evidence supporting their claim that Laetrile is effective.

A favorite gambit of all quacksters has been the charge that the scientific medical, governmental and ethical pharmaceutical "establishment" are in a conspiracy. This is clever because there is no way to disprove it. It is not possible to prove that something is not taking place secretly. The claim that several hundred thousand American and foreign physicians are in a world-wide conspiracy, although patently preposterous, is nevertheless persistently repeated by Laetrilists.

Lack of Scientific Publication

Good scientific evidence is published after competent review by scientists in recognized scientific journals, and presented at recognized scientific symposia. However, there are no reports in the recognized scientific publications that Laetrile "works". In contrast, Laetrile is propagandized by testimonials in popular journals, health cult magazines, on radio and television as well as by "word of mouth" in Laetrilist-organized meetings.

Claim Public Figures As Supporters

The Laetrilists claim prominent people, usually actors and politicians, as supporters. These individuals can be easily misled, as they are not trained or experienced in the natural history of cancer, the care of patients with cancer, or in scientific methodology.

Claims For Political Support (In Contrast to Medical Support)

The Laetrile proponents have failed to win acceptance from scientific medicine, but claim political success (17 states have legalized Laetrile). They claim that the medical "bureaucracy" has no right to withhold a patient's political right to "freedom of choice" of a treatment which the patient wants. Their political efforts do not address the merits of Laetrile as an efficacious drug, but rather the issue of "freedom of choice".

Claims (In Terms of Pseudo-Scientific Jargon) That the Method of Treatment Can Only Be Done by Themselves

In common with the supporters of other unproven cancer remedies, the Laetrilists stress that you "do not and cannot get results from Laetrile treatment unless you are a trained metabolic physician". The so-called "metabolic" physician is claimed to have special training in "metabolic therapy", and "holistic therapy" and "alternative therapy" - all phrases with a scientific ring to the unknowing, but pseudo-scientific nonsense to the informed.

The "Big" Lie

Taking the calculated risk that the audience is both gullible and uninformed, the quacks do not hesitate to reiterate "big" (but false) claims. Examples are: Laetrilists state that the Hunza people in Himalaya eat a high Laetrile - containing natural diet and that "there never has been a case of cancer in Hunza", conveniently ignoring reports to the exact contrary; Laetrilists claim that Israeli medicine has reported excellent results with Laetrile, despite sworn affidavits from Israel stating otherwise; Laetrilists continue to claim that Laetrile is a vitamin, despite their knowledge that all recognized nutritional experts state this claim to be false.

WHO MAKES, OR SHOULD MAKE, SCIENTIFIC POLICY?

The seventeen state legislatures that legalized Laetrile, did so despite the opposition of the scientific and medical "establishments". These decisions were in keeping with the longheld belief of the legitimate right of the public (through their politicians) to decide. However, the decision makes little sense.

Legislators must have confidence in the nation's scientific and medical institutions. If our experts are able, their judgment should be supported by the legislators. If not, our largely tax-financed scientific and medical institutions should be brought to the point where their expert's advice is respected. It makes no sense to train our nation's experts and then ignore their knowledge.

There is, of course, always the danger that government by experts would be government in the vested interests of experts. But politicians are also experts in their field, and could not the same concern be applied to them? The vested interest of the politicians is to be re-elected. Could not his decision therefore be based more on simply obtaining votes than on the overall merits of the problem? The political danger is that his decision may be founded on what is considered popular (or is made to appear popular by the organized pressures of special interest groups), rather than on nature's laws. In such event, the fallacy of a public policy so determined will soon be exposed, for nature will prevail.

These thoughts are not to be construed as advocating government by scientific experts. It is the people who should decide what is best for the general public, and not a single group. The best protection for a decision to be based on merit is through a well-informed public debate. That is a course that is dependent on the active participation of experts, but they must communicate their scientific facts in terms that are intelligible to laymen. A poorly informed electorate will make ill-advised recommendations to their legislators. If science believes its opinions should meet with acceptance, then they must counsel in plain clarifying words so easily understood that well-founded reason (based on merit and not on politics) will trimuph. There will be instances (unlike the Laetrile situation) where the experts themselves will not agree. At these times, sound regulatory policies certainly will be dependent on clear and adequate communication of all that is known if the general public's collective judgment is to reach valid decisions.

Human values are at risk in these matters. Society will have future choices regarding fraudulent drugs to make. Hopefully, this overview of unconventional (fraudulent) treatments of cancer will provide additional understanding and insight, and facilitate decisions consonant with the greatest protection of the public interest.

ACKNOWLEDGEMENTS

This research was supported in part by National Cancer Institute Contract NO1-CM-67081,and grants from the Chemotherapy Foundation of New York, the Burroughs Welcome Fund, and the American Cancer Society.

CONTRIBUTING AUTHORS

Joseph Aisner, M.D.
Associate Professor of Medicine
Head, Section of Medical Oncology
Baltimore Cancer Research Program
Division of Cancer Treatment
National Cancer Institute
Baltimore, Maryland 21201

Costan W. Berard, M.D.
Chief, Hematopathology Section
Laboratory of Pathology
National Cancer Institute
Bethesda, Maryland 20205

Raul C. Braylan, M.D.
Associate Professor of Pathology
University of Florida
College of Medicine
Gainesville, Florida 32611

Paul Chang, M.D.
Assistant Professor of Medicine
Senior Investigator
Baltimore Cancer Research Program
Division of Cancer Treatment
National Cancer Institute
Baltimore, Maryland 21201
Current address:
  Good Samaritan Hospital
  5601 Loch Raven Blvd.
  Baltimore, Maryland 21218

Marc Citron, M.D.
Fellow in Medical Oncology
Vincent T. Lombardi
  Cancer Research Center
Washington, D.C. 20007
Current address:
  29673 Farmbrook Villa Ct.
  Southfield, Michigan 48075

Charles H. Diggs, M.D.
Assistant Professor of Medicine
Senior Investigator
Baltimore Cancer Research Program
Division of Cancer Treatment
National Cancer Institute
Baltimore, Maryland 21201
Current address:
  1313 Fish-Hatchery Road
  Madison, Wisconsin 53715

Emil J. Freireich, M.D.
Professor of Medicine
Chief, Research Hematology
Head, Department of
  Developmental Therapeutics
M.D. Anderson Hospital
  and Tumor Institute
Houston, Texas 77030

John J. Gullo, M.D.
Fellow in Medical Oncology
Vincent T. Lombardi
  Cancer Research Center
Washington, D.C. 20007
Current address:
  Crouse-Irving Memorial
  Physicians Office Building
  Suite 302
  725 Irving Avenue
  Syracuse, New York 13210

Donald J. Higby, M.D.
Associate Chief Medicine A
Roswell Park Memorial Institute
Buffalo, New York 14263

Elaine S. Jaffe, M.D.
Senior Investigator
Laboratory of Pathology
National Cancer Institute
Bethesda, Maryland 20205

John Macdonald, M.D.
Assistant Professor of
  Medicine/Oncology
Vincent T. Lombardi
  Cancer Research Center
Washington, D.C. 20007
Currently:
  Chief, Chemotherapy Evaluation
    Program,
  Division of Cancer Treatment
  National Cancer Institute
  Bethesda, Maryland 20205

Richard G. Margolese, M.D.
Assistant Professor
McGill University
Director, Tumor Clinic
Jewish General Hospital
Montreal, Quebec, Canada

Daniel S. Martin, M.D.
Research Associate
Institute of Cancer Research
College of Physicians and Surgeons
Columbia University
New York, New York 10023

Alvin M. Mauer, M.D.
Medical Director
St. Jude Children's
  Research Hospital
Memphis, Tennessee 38105

Erlinds S. McCrea, M.D.
Assistant Professor
Department of Radiology
University of Maryland Hospital
Baltimore, Maryland 21201

Franco M. Muggia, M.D.
Associate Director,
Cancer Therapy Evaluation Program
Division of Cancer Treatment
National Cancer Institute
Bethesda, Maryland 20205
Currently:
  Director, Division of Oncology
  New York University Medical Center
  550 1st Avenue
  New York, New York 10016

Koji Nanba, M.D.
Chief, Department of Pathology
Kure Mutual Aide Hospital
Kure, Japan

Leonard R. Prosnitz, M.D.
Associate Professor of
  Therapeutic Radiology
Yale University School of Medicine
New Haven, Connecticut 06504

Marcel Rozencweig, M.D.
Special Assistant to the
  Associate Director
Cancer Therapy Evaluation Program
Division of Cancer Treatment
National Cancer Institute
Bethesda, Maryland 20205

Philip S. Schein, M.D.
Professor of Medicine
  and Pharmacology
Division of Medical Oncology
Georgetown University Hospital
Washington, D.C. 20007

Ralph Scott, M.D.
Professor and Chairman
Department of Radiation Therapy
University of Maryland Hospital
Baltimore, Maryland 21201

Patrick F. Sheedy, M.D.
Associate Professor of Radiology
  Mayo Graduate School of Medicine
Consultant in Radiology
  Mayo Clinic
Rochester, Minnesota 55901

Frederick P. Smith, M.D.
Assistant Professor
Department of Medical Oncology
Vincent T. Lombardi
  Cancer Research Center
Washington, D.C. 20007

David H. Stephens, M.D.
Assistant Professor of Radiology
Mayo Clinic
Rochester, Minnesota 55901

Wataru W. Sutow, M.D.
Chief, Division of Solid Tumors
Department of Pediatrics
Pediatrician & Professor of Pediatrics
M.D. Anderson Hospital
  and Tumor Institute
Houston, Texas 77030

Peter H. Wiernik, M.D.
Professor of Medicine
Chief, Clinical Oncology Branch
Acting Director
Baltimore Cancer Research Program
Division of Cancer Treatment
National Cancer Institute
Baltimore, Maryland 21201

John Wolfe, M.D.
Chief of Radiology
Hutzel Hospital
Detroit, Michigan 48201